From Hospital to Home Care

A Step by Step Guide to Providing Care to Patients Post Hospitalization

Kathy N. Johnson, PhD, CMC
James H. Johnson, PhD
Lily Sarafan, MS

The information contained in this book is intended to provide helpful and informative material on the subject addressed. It is not intended to serve as a replacement for professional medical advice. Any use of the information in this book is at the reader's discretion. The authors and publisher specifically disclaim any and all liability arising directly or indirectly from the use or application of any information contained in this book. A health care professional should be consulted regarding your specific situation.

All Rights Reserved. No part of this book may be used or reproduced in any matter without the written permission of the Publisher. Printed in the United States of America. For information address Home Care Press, 148 Hawthorne Avenue, Palo Alto, CA 94301.

ISBN 978-1-4675-0180-4

Copyright © 2012 Home Care Assistance, Inc.

ACKNOWLEDGMENTS

To the caregivers and health professionals who dedicate themselves to the wellbeing of patients everywhere.

TABLE OF CONTENTS

TABLE OF CONTENTS

TABLE OF CONTENTS

INTRODUCTION

When 62-year-old Elizabeth[1] drove herself to the emergency room on a cold, windy October night, she thought the pain in her abdomen was caused by a urinary tract infection. Her best friend thought it sounded more like gallstones, and her husband feared it was Appendicitis, so Elizabeth reluctantly agreed to leave the comfort of her home and get herself checked out by a doctor. She made her family and friends stay home.

Elizabeth never dreamed that she was suffering from late stage cervical cancer or that she would spend the next five years fighting—and ultimately losing the battle—for her life. During some of that time Elizabeth was in the hospital receiving various treatments, but she spent most of her days at home with the help of her family, a private-duty home care agency and finally, hospice.

Many people think of home care as something that applies only to frail elders; however, at least 65% of people who require home care receive this care after being discharged from an inpatient hospital stay.

Home care recipients can be people of any age who are suffering from a chronic or an acute disease, as well as people who are injured or who have had a surgical procedure. The common denominator among these people is that they all require extra assistance to stay in their homes.

---

[1] Name changed to protect her identity.

Whether your loved one is currently in the hospital or at home, this book will give you the tools and resources to meet the needs of your loved one throughout the transition from hospital to home. The book is separated into five sections and will explain many of the key issues of the post-hospitalization transition. In the first section, you will be introduced to the various needs of a recently discharged patient and the discharge process, including key players such as discharge planners, case managers and physical therapists, and the possible post-hospitalization settings. In the second section, you will learn about the most common concerns among post-discharge patients, such as comfort, safety and nutrition. The third section will review the nature of common medical problems across post-discharge patients, including pneumonia, joint replacement and cancer. In the fourth section you will receive an extensive review of the transition from hospital to home and advice on making the transition as seamless and comfortable as possible. The fifth and final section will provide you with a summary of the concepts covered throughout the book as well as an introduction to Home Care Assistance.

In the first chapter, you will read about a typical hospital discharge scenario and meet the members of the team who are responsible for helping the patient transition safely from hospital to home.

CHAPTER ONE
Discharge Planning in Action

It was just past 9:30 in the evening on a hot, July day. Jack, 78, and his wife Judy, 75, had just finished dinner and were sipping iced tea and watching television. Jack patted his wife's leg and went to bring some more ice from the kitchen. As he opened the freezer, something awful happened. He felt something in his left leg give way; the next thing he knew, he had fallen to the ground.

Judy heard him and rushed to his side. "Jack, are you okay?"

Embarrassment and intense pain made his tone harsher than normal. "Of course I am. I just lost my balance and fell. I'm fine." He tried to stand up, but his left leg refused to support him and he fell back on to the kitchen floor.

"I'm calling 911," Judy said firmly.

Jack winced. He did not like people making a fuss over him, but he had to admit that in this case, it was probably necessary.

As soon as the paramedics arrived, they exchanged glances over Jack's head.

"It may be a broken hip," one said, and the other nodded.

Utterly frustrated, Jack tried to tell them he didn't have time for a broken hip, he had a company to run, but the paramedics moved him gently onto a stretcher and rushed him to the hospital where their diagnosis was confirmed.

The next day, Jack went to surgery and the doctors replaced the shattered bone with a titanium rod. Jack was confused and disoriented when he got out of the surgery. He thought he was at home with his wife and did not understand why there were so many people in the house.

To Judy's relief, Jack's confusion cleared as the anesthetic wore off, but she was still worried about Jack coming home. There was no way to get into the house without going up a set of stairs and Jack wasn't even standing yet, let alone able to walk.

That afternoon, a nurse came into the room and introduced herself as the discharge planner. Jack was to be discharged, probably as early as the next day, and it was the discharge planner's job to make sure that Jack went to a setting where he would receive the appropriate care once he left the hospital.

Jack said he wanted to go home.

Judy forced herself to speak up, even though Jack glared at her. She pointed out that Jack couldn't even get into the house unless someone carried him. She was also concerned about her ability to assist him with things like bathing and dressing. Judy was a short woman who weighed 120 pounds. Jack stood over six feet tall and weighed 200 pounds.

The discharge planner listened and agreed with Judy that home was not an option, at least for the time being.

Jack, overcome with a sense of panic, announced "I may just kill myself if you put me in a nursing home."

The nurse called the physical and occupational therapists into the room and asked them about Jack's rehabilitation potential. They both thought it was excellent. Before the fracture he had been a strong, healthy man and though he was given to explosive outbursts, he didn't show any signs of dementia that could complicate a rehab program.

The discharge planner made the following suggestion: Suppose Jack went to a skilled rehabilitation facility located inside the hospital for a couple of weeks with the goal of getting strong enough to come home. Would that be an acceptable solution?

Judy breathed a sigh of relief when Jack reluctantly agreed that moving to a rehabilitation unit was probably his best option. He just wanted to be sure his Medicare[2] would cover it.

The discharge planner spoke to the person in charge of patient accounts, who said that Jack's Medicare and Medicaid policies would cover the cost in full.

Later, the doctor phoned the discharge planner to tell her he had read the details of Jack's post-hospitalization care and was in agreement with the plan.

---

[2] Government health benefit for seniors. For more information on U.S. benefits, visit medicare.gov. For more information on Canadian benefits, visit www.hc-sc.gc.ca

That evening, a social worker came in to talk with Jack. She was concerned that he had threatened suicide. Embarrassed, Jack told her he hadn't meant it. He was just frustrated and worried that he would never be able to go home again. As he spoke, his eyes filled with tears.

The social worker comforted him and reassured him that his good health before the fracture would work in his favor. She told him that she had seen many of people in worse shape than him leave rehab and go home. She also reminded him that he could trust his "new" hip. Titanium does not shatter or buckle like bone. Jack felt better and slept well that night.

The next day he went to the rehabilitation unit, where he stayed for almost three weeks. By the time he left, he was moving around with a walker and able to climb a few stairs which meant that he could get into his home. He could also dress and bathe himself, as long as someone stood nearby to assist if necessary.

At home, Jack's progress continued with the help of family. Both of his sons came to visit regularly to help their mother with the care Jack still needed. It wasn't long before they decided they could benefit from additional help. The physically demanding tasks required as part of Jack's rehabilitation were exhausting and overwhelming for Judy. Her sons also began to sense the emotional toll often associated with providing personal hygiene and care for a parent who had previously been strong and independent. They discussed private duty home care and agreed that this would be a great option to provide respite for the family. A screened and trained caregiver, Shanna, came to the house three days a week for six hours at a time. During these visits, Shanna assisted Jack with his bathing, grooming and physical therapy exercises, prepared nutritious meals and, most important, relieved Judy of her sense of guilt when she ran errands or attended social functions.

After six weeks, Jack was able to drive his car to and from work. A week after that, he traded his walker for a cane, and two weeks later, he stopped using the cane altogether. Six months out from the fracture, he was walking almost normally again.

Today, Jack and his family are relieved and thankful.

"Looking back, it's almost like it was just a bad dream," Judy says.

Jack admits that he still carries a few emotional scars in addition to the physical ones. He's very apprehensive about going into the kitchen by himself, for instance. Where once he walked confidently, knowing his body would do what it was supposed to do, he now walks slowly, testing his weight on each foot. He is afraid of another fall, but is relieved to be home with his family. He's trying to remain positive about the future.

CHAPTER TWO
The Who's Who of Hospital Discharge

In the last chapter, you were able to witness discharge planning taking place at a breakneck speed. Now, let's roll the tape back and take a look at the many people who play a role in the planning process.

Patient

The first and most important person in the discharge planning process is the patient. As long as he is mentally capable, the patient has the right to discharge into any situation at all, even one that his care team deems unsafe. The patient may also discharge himself against medical advice. Most patients, however, want to go into the safest and most supportive environment possible, so they work with the planning team, offering valuable insights into what they will need to make a smooth and efficient transition home.

Family Members/Caregivers

Family members and caregivers are a vital part of the discharge planning process because they are the ones who will help manage the patient's care in the home or wherever else the patient may go. Every discharge planner knows all too well that if the family members and caregivers don't buy into a discharge plan, that plan will probably not succeed.

This is illustrated clearly in the case of Dan and Luke[3]. Dan, an 86-year-old man, was a serious alcoholic who had been drinking steadily since he was in his early twenties. His cognition was severely compromised. In addition, he suffered from lung disease and diabetic neuropathy. He had an apartment attached to the house of his son, Luke, and sometimes became confused at night and stumbled around the small space, often falling or scraping and bruising himself against doorways. Sometimes his falls necessitated a hospital stay.

It was clear to all the healthcare professionals who worked with Dan that his current living arrangement was not safe. Even Dan admitted he was often lonely and frightened while his son was at work. Luke, however, believed that putting his father in a nursing facility would be an act of betrayal.

Only after Dan stumbled outside one night, tumbled down the porch steps, hit his head and remained unconscious on the ground all night, was Luke willing to agree that his father probably needed more help than he could provide on his own. Shaken after seeing Dan lying on the ground, Luke quickly hired live-in care from Home Care Assistance to provide around the clock support for his father. The two caregivers who provided 24/7 care for Dan stayed with him for seven years until Dan passed away. Luke still stays in touch with his father's caregivers who helped him live happily and safely where he most wanted to be, home.

Physician

Next to the patient, the physician is the team member who has the most input. The physician frequently makes recommendations

---

[3] Names changed to protect their privacy.

about the best place for the patient to recuperate and authorizes the final discharge plans. If the physician disagrees with a team's plan, the team must start over and develop a plan more in line with the physician's thinking. The physician is also responsible for prescribing discharge medications which can have a direct bearing on the patient's comfort and mood.

The physician has the same ultimate goal as the patient: the patient's physical and mental wellbeing. Further, given new standards for many hospitals that closely monitor readmission rates, the physician wants to ensure that the patient is taken care of post-discharge in order to avoid readmission.

The physician that the patient sees in the hospital is often different from the patient's personal or primary care physician. As the patient's personal doctor may not see the patient during the hospital admission, and plays little to no role in discharge planning, there can be a gap in communication that occurs among the primary care physician and other key players on the team. If it is possible to involve the patient's personal physician at this stage, it can be very helpful to include any suggestions or notes to the discharge planners.

Nurse(s)

The nurses who have taken care of the patient day in and day out are an extremely valuable resource during the discharge planning process. They are able to comment, for instance, on the patient's mental status, stamina and ability and willingness to follow directions. They can also discuss the patient's mood and cognitive status and bring potential problems to the attention of the team.

Often, nurses are the first people to notice depression and mild cognitive impairment, both of which are important factors to consider when creating a patient's discharge plan. Again, communication is key and the nurses will have extremely valuable input to share with the discharge team.

Discharge Planner

The discharge planner is usually a nurse, though he or she may also be a social worker. It is their job to coordinate all the resources to get the patient out of the hospital as soon as possible. The discharge planner faces a lot of pressure in this job. They answer to the utilization committee, which determines when a patient's insurance will stop covering his stay in the hospital. Often, the utilization committee pressures the discharge planner to arrange quick discharges for patients with complex social situations.

He or she may also face pressure from a family who doesn't want the patient discharged from the hospital so quickly.

The discharge planner wears several hats. They have to consider what is cost-effective for the hospital while also considering the family's wishes and the wellbeing of the patient. He or she must play the roles of negotiator, counselor, persuader and sometimes drill sergeant. The discharge planner must also maintain good relationships with other community agencies such as rehabilitation hospitals, nursing facilities, hospices and home health companies.

Social Worker

A social worker may at times fill the discharge planning role. Usually, though, the social worker has three chief three responsibilities.

First, she must assess the patient for psychosocial factors that could impact discharge plans. For example, if the social worker discovers that the patient is living with an abusive spouse or facing some other type of harm at home, it is her job to coordinate with the discharge planner to make sure the patient goes to a safe environment after discharge. When patients threaten to harm themselves, the social worker is typically called in to assess the patient's risk of suicide.

Second, the social worker helps to connect families with relevant community resources. She may set up home-delivered meals, for instance, or give the patient referrals to a private duty home care company for extra care at home. If the family can't come to an agreement on certain aspects of the patient's care, the responsibility often falls to the social worker to set up a meeting with the physician to try to get everyone on the same page.

Third, the social worker is available to patients and their families for emotional support and guidance.

Skilled Therapists – OT/PT/ST

Occupational therapists, physical therapists and speech therapists can also play a role in the discharge planning process by communicating the patient's capabilities and deficits to the discharge planner. As you may remember in the last chapter, the discharge planner did not place going to a rehabilitation unit on the table as an option until after she had spoken with the skilled therapists and learned that they considered Jack an "excellent" rehab candidate.

The skilled therapists can also help train family members about the types of physical care that the patient needs and how the family can best assist.

Geriatric Care Manager

Geriatric care managers are individuals who have been professionally trained to work with patients and their families to help the patient reach and maintain his or her highest level of functioning. The geriatric care manager usually has a background in one of the health and/or helping professions such as gerontology, nursing, social work, or psychology. He or she works to coordinate services for the patient. If the patient's family is out of town or otherwise unable to participate in their loved one's care, the geriatric care manager acts as a liaison between the different agencies providing services to the patient and the often overwhelmed family members.

Many geriatric care managers maintain independent businesses in the community. These care managers become a part of the discharge planning process when they are hired by the patient's family.

Geriatric care managers usually do a comprehensive assessment of the patient, noting his or her physical, social and emotional strengths and weaknesses. They also talk to family members and friends about their concerns. The care manager then creates a care plan reflecting the best environment for the patient as well as the services the patient needs to best function in that environment. If the family supports the care plan, the care manager coordinates the necessary services.

Resource Corner: If you believe your loved one could benefit from the advocacy of a geriatric care manager, visit the National Association of Professional Geriatric Care Manager (NAPGCM) website at **www.caremanager.org**. The organization serves the United States and Canada.

Home Health Care Agency

The days when people could spend months leisurely recuperating in a hospital are long past. And that's probably a good thing. As one physician commented while talking about hospital-acquired infections, "A hospital is the worst place in the world to be if you're sick."

For better or for worse, the trend now is to rush patients out of the hospital as soon as possible, even if they continue to have skilled needs such as requiring dressing changes, needing IV medications or experiencing serious mobility problems. When this occurs, a home health care agency is included in the discharge planning process. Some home health care agencies are owned and operated by the hospital; others are community based. In every case, it is the right of the patient and family members to select the agency they prefer to provide home health care.

14

Home health care agencies are covered by Medicare to help patients who need the intermittent skilled services of a nurse, physical therapist, occupational therapist, or speech therapist. The length of time a home health care agency provides services is usually fairly short, on the order of one to two hours per day for 30 days or less.

Home Care Agency

For many patients, completing basic day-to-day activities is the most daunting aspect of leaving the hospital. Home care agencies are a resource that can provide assistance with what are termed activities of daily living (ADLs), such as bathing, grooming, dressing, light housekeeping and meal preparation. Caregivers from home care agencies can also assist with running errands, companionship throughout the recovery process, support through rehabilitation exercises or simply keeping a sharp eye on a patient who poses a significant fall risk.

Home care, also known as private duty care, is typically paid for out of pocket. Most long term care insurance plans will also cover home care.

Resource Corner: Visit Home Care Assistance at **www.HomeCareAssistance.com** to learn more about in-home care services, find a home care location near you and subscribe to educational content through the blog and e-newsletter.

Hospice

If a patient is terminally ill, with a prognosis of six months or fewer left to live, and if the patient has exhausted all the treatments available or simply declines further treatment, hospice will probably be asked to participate in the discharge planning process. Like home health care, hospice is a Medicare benefit. Many hospitals have their own hospice programs and there are also many independent hospice programs in the community. The patient and his or her family, of course, have the right to choose which hospice they would like to receive care from.

While home health care usually focuses on a cure, or at least stabilization, hospice, also sometimes referred to as palliative care, focuses on quality of life for patients with life-limiting conditions. Rather than trying to cure the underlying disease, hospice nurses provide aggressive symptom management with the goal of keeping the patient as comfortable and as mobile as possible for as long as possible.

Although the medical community is becoming more accepting of hospice, there are still some physicians who feel strongly that a hospice referral is synonymous with "giving up." Other doctors simply aren't sure how to broach the topic with patients and their families.

Resource Corner: If your loved one has a limited life expectancy and is no longer undergoing treatment for his or her illness, ask the doctor if your loved one is an appropriate candidate for hospice services. You can also contact a local care manager at **caremanager.org** to request recommendations for hospice organizations.

The disciplines listed above describe the main players in getting your loved one safely out of the hospital with a plan to ensure continued care. Of course, most people want their loved ones to be discharged directly back home; however, the discharge planning team may suggest an alternate setting or facility for an interim period.

CHAPTER THREE
Helping the Discharge Planner

As discussed in the last chapter, the discharge planner is responsible for coordinating all aspects of the discharge. In doing so, he or she relies heavily on information provided by the hospital team, and even more heavily on information provided by the hospitalized person's significant other, family, or friends.

Maryanne Reimer, Nurse Practitioner, who is involved in discharge planning at the Frederick Memorial Hospital, said that the first two things she always addresses are whether or not there is support in the home, and whether or not the home is a safe environment. In looking at safety, Reimer carefully assesses all aspects of the home environment, from throw rugs that could get caught under the patient's feet and cause a fall to rambunctious animals who might inadvertently trip their owners.

Debra Stang, LCSW, who performed hospital discharge planning at a community hospital, adds that an important safety consideration is who else is in the home with the patient. Providing a harrowing example, Stang describes, "If you're sending a dying patient home on heavy doses of pain medication," she says, "you want to make sure that the son who just got out of prison on a drug dealing charge will not be allowed in the home unsupervised."

Another important aspect of safety planning is ensuring that the patient always has a way to call for help by ringing a bell, carrying a cell phone at all times or wearing a personal medical alarm.

Maryanne Reimer explains that it makes the hospital discharge planner's job much easier if the family has had some honest talks before a crisis or hospitalization takes place. "Discharge planning," she says, "actually begins with an elderly couple talking to their family about what to do if something happens to Grandpa." Families that have plans in place tend to be much more successful in bringing their loved ones home than families who passively leave discharge arrangements to the hospital. "The public," Reimer reflects, is often under the impression that the hospital or the doctor will take care of everything and that they have no obligation to be prepared for health-related events." Indeed, family members often do not want to think about a loved one needing hospitalization, so discharge planning is not a topic of discussion until after the fact.

Debra Stang recalls, "If a doctor complained to me that a family was being a real pain in the neck with too many questions, I figured I was going to get along with them just fine. At least they were taking an active role in asking questions and making plans. You can't be passive about something as important as your loved one's care after hospitalization."

As important as the family's role is—and it is vital—the hospital, too, plays an important role in the discharge process. For example, having updated and accurate insurance information is one way the patient accounts department can facilitate next steps for the discharge planner in developing a post-hospitalization plan for the patient.

Doctors also play an important role in helping with the discharge process. Maryanne Reimer reports frustration with individuals on the discharge planning team who don't know what services are available but promise patients the impossible anyway. If someone, for instance, has said that a patient can have a visiting nurse come twice a day, but the discharge planner finds that the patient lacks the insurance or financial wherewithal to support this level of care, the family may blame the discharge planner, when in reality, their insurance plan only covers two nursing visits a week.

If your loved one is hospitalized, and you have been told about available services that seem too good to be true, verify the statements with your discharge planner, or ask to speak directly to the community agency that will be providing those services. While it is understandably an upsetting situation to learn that the services you were promised are not available after all, it is important to keep in mind that there are many players in the discharge process who may have different levels of knowledge about what programs and levels of assistance are actually available. Typically, your best resources are the discharge planners and social workers who will have the most hands-on experience with these issues.

Doctors can also help by writing comprehensive and timely discharge orders and by giving the discharge planner a "heads up" when they think a discharge will soon be taking place. A variety of factors can often make this impossible, however, and there may be situations where discharge nurses are informed only right before the discharge is to take place. In these situations, it can become a struggle to get a plan together that will ensure patient safety over the coming days and weeks.

Another way that you, the family members, can help discharge planners is to take action quickly if you are asked to do so. If a discharge planner meets with you on Tuesday, for instance, and asks you to start looking at skilled nursing facilities where your loved one can recuperate, start looking immediately. That way, if your loved one is discharged quickly and without much warning, the discharge planner already knows which facilities you prefer and will have a much easier time arranging the transfer.

One thing that is important for you to remember is that the discharge planner can make all the arrangements he or she wants, but ultimately the final call is left to the patient who is capacitated, that is, a patient who is alert, oriented and able to make reasonable decisions, While the family members may not like the decision that the patient makes, it is her right as a patient to choose where she wants to go following discharge.

Debra Stang recalls a time, for instance, when she worked with a young woman who had suffered a bad fall, fracturing both legs. The doctors wanted her to go to a nursing facility to recuperate. The patient, however, had different ideas. Her grandmother had died in a nursing home and she was "scared to death" of such places.

After a lot of discussion with the patient, the family, the patient's insurance company and the doctors, the group all agreed on discharging the patient to the home of an aunt who was a licensed nurse practitioner. The aunt's home had only one story, so it was well-suited for a wheelchair. The insurance company, relieved that they would not have to cover a nursing home bill, agreed to waive the co-pay on the equipment the patient needed and also approved two months of physical therapy visits in the home. This was a discharge plan with which the patient could happily agree.

A few months later, the patient's mother called to let Debra know that everything went as planned and that her daughter was walking with the assistance of a walker. The patient was expected to make a full recovery.

Your loved one's wishes matter. Your wishes also matter. If you don't like the direction a discharge planner is taking, speak up and ask what other options are available, otherwise you and your loved one may not get exactly what you want. For instance, due to the fact that her patient's mother lived in an old home with narrow staircases, Debra's patient had to go to an aunt's home rather than back to her mother's home, but at least she avoided the frightening idea of a nursing home.

If you're trying to bring your loved one home, you may need to get creative and involve several members of the family. For instance, if your father has suffered a stroke and the doctor tells your mother he can't be alone, perhaps each child in the family could volunteer to spend an evening or two with their father to give their mother respite. Another option is hiring a caregiver from a reputable private duty home care agency, or recruiting members from your church or from your neighborhood to help.

The more closely you work with the discharge planner, the more likely it is that you will be pleased with the outcome.

CHAPTER FOUR
Where Do Discharged Patients Go?

Most discharged patients want nothing more than to go home, but home isn't always a realistic option. Newly discharged patients may require more care than their family can provide. If paying for private duty care isn't an option, the patient may have no choice but to go to a rehabilitation facility or nursing home in an effort to get stronger.

Some patients can't go home because of physical or functional barriers. Remember Jack in Chapter One who wasn't able to climb the stairs to get into his home?

Still others can't go home because they live with a family member who is abusive or neglectful. If a person, especially a child or an elderly person suffering from confusion, comes to the hospital with unexplained injuries the hospital staff will very likely notify the police or child/adult protective services. If these entities investigate and agree that the injuries are suspicious for abuse, the patient will almost always be discharged to an alternate location.

Some of the most common discharge locations are discussed below:

Skilled Nursing Facility

The Medicare benefit pays for up to 100 days of rehabilitation and skilled nursing care in a skilled nursing facility (often called a nursing home). The first 20 days are covered in full by Medicare and the next 80 involve a copay which may be covered by secondary insurance. In order to remain eligible for Medicare, the person must show that he is making progress in therapy, or that his condition is unstable enough to require around the clock skilled nursing.

As the patient nears the end of her 100 days, or if she becomes ineligible for further services (e.g. no progress in therapy, no continued skilled nursing needs), the family needs to request a meeting with the rehabilitation team, the head nurse of the unit and the patient's social worker to discuss options.

For most people it comes down to two choices: (1) return to their own home or the home of a relative when their Medicare coverage ends or (2) remain in a facility setting as a "private pay" resident. If the person does not have the money to pay privately for ongoing facility care, he or she will have to apply for the state's medical assistance program, generally called Medicaid. Medicaid will cover long-term room and board in a facility for as long as a doctor deems it necessary.

Rehabilitation Facility

A rehabilitation facility is as one patient put it, "like a nursing home rehabilitation on steroids." A rehabilitation facility can be located in a wing of the hospital or it can be a stand-alone facility.

Rehabilitation facilities generally accept patients with a good chance of returning to the community when rehab is completed.

During a typical rehab stay, a patient may be put through several hours of work with a physical, occupational, or speech therapist as well as given exercises to do independently.

Patients usually dress in their own clothing and are encouraged to eat meals together and socialize so they can support each other. In the best case scenario, this creates a community environment that enables the patient to feel supported as she or he recovers.

Rehabilitation usually lasts only a few weeks, and at the end of that time, the patient is usually able to return to her own home or the home of a relative who will assist with her care.

Hospice

Some people with a life-limiting illness come into the hospital due to a "pain emergency." If that person's pain or other unpleasant symptoms cannot be controlled outside of the hospital setting, inpatient hospice may be suggested. In general, inpatient hospices take two types of patients: patients whom they feel only have a few days left to live and patients who cannot be made comfortable at home.

If your loved one falls into the first group, the goal is to create a setting for your loved to pass peacefully in the inpatient hospice unit. Inpatient hospices are very understanding and not only permit, but encourage families to spend as much time as possible with the dying patient. They many times also provide bereavement and support services to family members after the patient has passed.

If your loved one falls into the second group, the job of the hospice unit will be to aggressively manage comfort. The focus becomes quality of life and ensuring that the patient is as comfortable as possible. For instance, the hospice team might recommend that your loved one get a pain pump so she can receive medications intravenously in small, scheduled doses. The expectation is that the hospice team will be able to control the pain or other distressing symptoms, and that the patient will then be discharged home where she can be followed by an outpatient hospice team.

The Community (Home)

The goal of most hospitalized patients is to leave the institutional setting, whether that means returning to their own homes or going to the homes of friends or family members to recuperate.

The patient who returns to the community has a number of resources to maintain comfort and support.

Medical Equipment. Medicare and most other insurance companies cover at least a portion of the bill for the medical equipment your loved one needs to safely function at home. Items that are covered may include a wheelchair, a hospital bed, an oxygen concentrator, a walker, or a cane. Please note that insurance companies typically do not cover "non-medical" items, such as a reclining chair that lifts to make standing easier. If you need medical equipment but do not have insurance that will cover the equipment, let your social worker know as soon as possible. She or he may be able to refer you to a loan center or a warehouse where you can get the equipment you need less expensively.

Home Health Care. Home health care is a benefit typically covered under Medicare. This benefit can only be used by patients who require intermittent skilled care—care that must be provided by a nurse or a licensed therapist. Nursing and/or therapy visits are usually scheduled one to three times per week and the patient is usually discharged from the program within a few weeks as his skilled needs dissipate.

Hospice. Hospice programs provide palliative care to patients with a terminal illness. In order to qualify for hospice, a patient can no longer be undergoing curative treatment, and a doctor must certify that the patient's life expectancy is six months or less. Some hospices have a hospice house where a patient can go when she has symptoms that cannot be controlled at home or when she is within a few days of death. Most hospices are set up to make home visits to patients in need. Hospice is very focused on relieving and preventing suffering. If your loved one receives hospice care, he will have a nurse/case manager who coordinates care with the patient, family, doctor and the rest of the hospice team, usually comprised of a licensed nurse practitioner, social worker, chaplain and a home health aide to assist with activities such as bathing, dressing, light housekeeping and preparing simple meals. Most patients receive hospice services until they pass or until their condition stabilizes and their doctor believes that their condition has improved to the point where their life expectancy is beyond six months.

Private Duty Home Care Company. A private duty home care company provides what is called non-medical care. This is routine care that the patient needs to remain at home. A caregiver helps the patient with bathing or showering, getting dressed in the morning and ready for bed at night, brushing hair, shaving, running errands, making phone calls, light housekeeping and additional activities of daily living as required. Medicare and most health insurance plans do not pay for private duty care. Typically, if your loved one requires private duty assistance, he is likely to have to pay out of pocket for at least a portion of the services received. Still, there are a number of options that may help finance non-medical in-home care. If your loved one has long term care insurance, private duty care in the home may be a covered benefit. There are also programs available for those with low income and very few assets. Finally, if your loved one is a veteran or spouse of a veteran, she or he may be eligible for financial assistance for home care from a veteran's pension fund.

Geriatric Care Manager. A geriatric care manager is a person familiar with the healthcare field and with the special needs of aging and disabled clients. Most geriatric care managers have a background in nursing, psychology, gerontology or social work. A geriatric care manager can coordinate and manage your loved one's care if you live out of town or if you are simply too overwhelmed to take it on. Services that a geriatric care manager can provide include assessing the patient to determine her needs and wishes, selecting the appropriate agency to provide services in the home, provide crisis intervention, assist with legal and financial matters and provide advocacy and emotional support for you and your loved one.

Safety Devices. If your loved one is frail and lives alone, you might want to consider getting her a personal medical alarm. The alarm consists of a transmission box that is hooked into the telephone and has a wireless alarm button that the patient wears as a bracelet or necklace. If your loved one has a fall, he or she can push the button to summon help.

You may also need to consider safety devices if you are bringing a patient with dementia into your home. Since patients with cognitive impairments tend to wander, it is smart to invest in door alarms for all of the outside doors. A baby monitor is also useful at night because it can alert you if your loved one gets out of bed and starts wandering around the house. Other measures you might want to consider include disabling the stove and oven and checking your hot water thermostat to make sure the temperature does not get too high. One frustrated caregiver described having a loved one with Alzheimer's in the home: "It's like sharing your home with someone who has the size and strength of an adult and the judgment of a two-year-old."

These suggestions are designed to help you get your loved one home from the hospital safely. The next chapters explore issues and challenges people experience upon discharge from the hospital setting and how best to deal with these issues.

CHAPTER FIVE
Post-Discharge Concerns: Pain

Depending on why your loved one went into the hospital, pain management may be a concern for her when she comes home. This is especially true if she was hospitalized due to an accident or injury, if she underwent surgery while in the hospital, or if she has been diagnosed with a terminal illness that causes pain. Of course, your loved one may suffer from other types of pain that have nothing to do with her hospitalization. For instance, she may suffer from chronic joint pain due to arthritis or back pain caused by a long-ago car accident.

There are individual differences in the way people experience pain and people will have varying pain thresholds. While some people have an incredibly high tolerance for pain and seem to barely notice it, others may be extremely bothered by even a mild headache. Communication is key in understanding how bothersome the pain is for your loved one. A useful tactic that many nurses use in hospital emergency rooms is to ask the individual to rate the pain intensity on a scale from 1 to 10, one being no pain and 10 being the worst pain the person has ever felt.

If you suspect your loved one will have pain or discomfort at home, discuss this problem with the hospital discharge planner and with the physician. Although leading health accreditation bodies like the Canadian Council on Health Services Accreditation (CCHSA-Canada) and the Joint Commission on Accreditation of Healthcare Organizations (JCAHO-USA) have made treating pain a priority, defining it as the "fifth vital sign," doctors may be reluctant to adequately treat pain for many reasons. The chief one is that the most powerful pain relievers are opioids, which can be addictive if misused. Another reason is that pain medications can cause side effects that are bothersome, including constipation and drowsiness. From the patients' side, the patient may not always report the pain she is experiencing to the physician for fear that treating the pain will detract from treating "more important" medical concerns.

If the patient is uncomfortable and you do not feel that the medical team overseeing the care is taking the pain seriously or treating it as aggressively as they should be, ask for a referral to the palliative care team if the patient is still in the hospital, or to a pain management clinic if he or she has already been discharged.

Non-Prescription Remedies

There are many medications that can be used to manage pain and many of them are available over the counter. Over the counter medications include:

Acetaminophen. Acetaminophen, better known as Tylenol, treats fever and pain. It does not, however, treat inflammation.

NSAIDs. Nonsteroidal Anti-Inflammatory Drugs such as aspirin, ibuprofen, and Aleve treat both pain and inflammation and are also used to lower fever. NSAIDs are effective pain medications, but they can be very hard on the stomach. They also have blood-thinning properties.

Topical Creams. Topical creams such as Aspercreme and Ben-Gay provide temporary relief for sore muscles and mild to moderate pain caused by arthritis.

Do not give your loved one any of these medications unless you have first discussed it with her doctor to make sure there are no counter-indications. A man with a history of stomach ulcers, for instance, is not a good candidate for long-term use of NSAIDS.

In addition to medications, there are some steps you can take at home that may help relieve your loved one's pain. Applying an icepack or a heated towel to the painful area can ease discomfort following an injury. If your loved one is bed bound, helping her to change positions in the bed can also bring some relief. Another technique is distraction. Talk to your loved one about something not related to pain or medical issues. Get her interested in listening to a favorite song, watching a show or a sporting event on television, stroking a pet, or giving you advice on something on which she considers herself an expert.

You will be able to better help your loved one if you stay calm. Even if you're frustrated at the medical team or extremely upset that your loved one is in pain, offering reassurance in a calm, confident voice can help ease your loved one's nerves.

These may be only stop-gap measures, but they can help to relieve pain while you are working to get stronger pain-relieving measures in place. Discuss prescription medications with the patient's physician.

What to Do in the Event of a Pain Crisis

If your loved one is experiencing severe pain, known to healthcare professionals as a pain crisis, place an immediate call to her doctor, home health nurse, or hospice nurse. If your patient has home health or hospice services, the nurses will probably be able to talk to the doctor and handle the crisis in the home. They may do this by starting your loved one on a new pain medication, changing a pain medication currently in place, or giving a larger dosage of the medication your loved one is currently using.

If your loved one is not signed up with home health or hospice, the doctor will probably suggest transporting her to the nearest emergency room so that her pain can be assessed and managed. Your loved one may be admitted to the hospital where she can receive medications intravenously. Another possibility is that your loved one will require a pain pump which is placed under the skin and regularly releases small doses of opioids.

Pain emergencies are frightening for the patient and extremely disturbing to families, but the good news is that most types of pain, even the types that result from metastatic cancer, are treatable. Your loved one can come through this crisis and do well at home once the appropriate pain management plan is set into motion.

CHAPTER SIX
Post-Discharge Concerns: Safety at Home

One of the hospital discharge team's chief concerns is the patient's safety in the home setting. Four of the main areas of concern include falls, fires and burns, proper use of medication and the risk of the patient becoming confused and wandering away, also known as elopement.

Falls

When your loved one comes home from the hospital, he may still be feeling the effects of an anesthetic if he underwent a surgical procedure. If he is on medication for pain or anxiety, that can also contribute to him being unsteady on his feet. Finally, if your loved one's diagnosis includes Parkinson's or Alzheimer's, he may walk with a shuffling, uncertain gait that puts him at risk for tripping over things on the floor.

The first thing you can do to prevent falls is take a quick tour and observe your home. Are the major walkways clear of towels, clothes, books, toys or any other item that could cause your loved one to trip or stumble? Enlist your family, especially your children, in the task of clearing the walkways every single day. Not only will your house be neater, but your children can feel a sense of pride that they are doing something to help your loved one.

There a number of common household items that should be especially heeded as they contribute most frequently to falls.

Throw rugs pose a safety concern for someone who is a fall risk. Even though they may be attractive, it's just too easy for someone walking with an unsteady gait to get his feet tangled up in them and take a fall.

After clearing your home of any throw rugs, check your electrical cords. Make sure they do not stretch across the hallways, doorways, or any other path that your loved one routinely takes through the house. If your loved one comes home wearing an oxygen mask, you will want to keep an eye on the long pieces of tubing to make sure they are not coiling near your loved one's feet. People who are not used to wearing oxygen masks often trip and fall over the unfamiliar tubing.

Next, the focus should be shifted to the bathroom. Installing grab bars by the toilet and in the shower so that your loved one has something to hang on to as he takes care of personal hygiene is an excellent and often necessary safety precaution. Placing a slip-free mat in the shower is also a good idea and will prevent your loved one from slipping.

The lighting should also be checked in each room that your loved one frequents to ensure that it is adequate. People with poor eyesight often trip over items on the floor or walk into furniture because they simply can't see objects in front of them.

People who are considered at high risk for falling are generally discharged from the hospital with an assistive device, like a walker or a cane. If your loved one comes home with such a device, make sure he uses it. People often resist the use of assistive equipment, claiming they aren't at risk for falling and don't need assistance. Be understanding with your loved one, but be firm. Emphasize that the assistive equipment was recommended by the physician who considered it a necessity. Many older adults view doctors as authority figures and will heed the words of physicians more closely. It's also a good technique to make the doctor the "heavy" so your loved one doesn't become angry with you.

Finally, if your loved one will be left alone in the house, rent or buy a personal medical alarm so that he can push a button and summon help in the event of a fall or other emergency. Many people suffer less from the fall itself than they do from the effects of lying on the ground for hours, waiting to be rescued.

Fires/Burns

There are many causes contributing to household fires, but an all too common scenario often involves someone with dementia or mild cognitive impairment misusing kitchen equipment. If your loved one is confused, it's a wise idea to disconnect ovens, stovetops and even the microwave. Social worker Debra Stang recalls working with a confused patient who put all of his important documents in the microwave and set the timer for five minutes. Only the fortuitous diligence of his wife prevented a house fire.

If your loved one uses oxygen, make sure he knows that he absolutely, positively cannot smoke while wearing his nasal cannula or oxygen mask. If he insists on smoking, turn off the concentrator and move the concentrator and tubing into another room while your loved one smokes.

Another common cause of household fires is lit cigarettes falling on the ground when the smoker falls asleep while smoking. In situations where a loved one suffers from confusion, you may want to set a rule that he can only smoke during the day while someone is there to watch over him. Some medical equipment companies also sell "smoking aprons," a flame-retardant blanket that goes over your loved one's lap. If he falls asleep and drops the cigarette on the apron, no harm is done.

As a basic safety precaution, it's also a good idea to check all of your electrical wiring and arrange for any wiring that is frayed or worn to be replaced. Finally, you should have at least one smoke detector for every floor of your house. If you live in a large house with a lot of open spaces, you may need more than one smoke detector per floor. Contact your local fire department for help obtaining and installing trustworthy smoke detectors.

People with cognitive impairment are also at risk for burns from hot water. Therefore, if your loved one has dementia, turn the water thermostat down so that the water cannot reach temperatures hot enough to scald. It's also a good idea to remove any space heaters. Your loved one may touch the space heater, not knowing what it is, or he may stumble and fall into it, resulting in a painful burn.

Medication Safety

Keeping a list of your loved one's medications handy is always important. Ideally, you should know the name of each medication, its indication, the correct dosage and when your loved one needs to take it. If you aren't sure about some of the medications that your loved one is taking, call his doctor, the pharmacy or the home health or hospice nurse for further information as it may be unnecessary or have the potential to interact adversely with other medications.

Medications should be stored in their original containers. A pillbox marked with the days of the week is also an acceptable storage place if it helps you and your loved one keep track of when the medicine should be taken.

If your loved one is confused, do not give him access to his medication, as he may unintentionally take additional dosage. You should also keep all medications out of the reach of children.

Wandering/Elopement

Wandering and elopement (leaving the house unobserved) are very real and dangerous risks for people with impaired memory. The wife of one patient talks about how her husband, who suffered from Alzheimer's, always used to go out to get the morning paper. One day he picked up the paper from the sidewalk, turned, and could not remember which house he lived in. Luckily, he knocked on the door of a neighbor who recognized him and brought him safely home, but after that, his wife always accompanied him when he went outside.

There are several ways to prevent your loved one leaving the home without your knowledge. One is to install door alarms which make a loud, unpleasant noise whenever the door is opened without proper authorization. Not only will the alarm alert you that someone is exiting, it may also startle your loved one away from the door.

Another way to reduce the risk of wandering is to install tricky locks well above or below eye level on doors leading to the outside. However, one serious risk with this method that should be assessed is the potential for your loved one to become trapped inside the home if there is a fire or other emergency.

One woman whose husband had been a by-the-rules guy all his life simply created large signs that read, "STOP! DO NOT ENTER!" to place on the doors. Her husband grumbled about the restrictions, but he never attempted to open a door with a sign on it.

Resource Corner: If your loved one is at risk of wandering, consider enrolling him with a local Safe Return Program. These programs work closely with police to make every effort to return wandering patients to their homes as soon as possible. For more information, contact your local Alzheimer's Association.

This chapter examined some threats to your loved one's physical wellbeing and offered some precautionary tips. The next chapter discusses the psychological effects your loved one may experience after a hospitalization.

CHAPTER SEVEN
Post-Discharge Concerns: Psychology

A person who has been hospitalized and has returned home may experience a wide range of emotions, both positive and negative. Someone whose hospital stay was relatively short and who anticipates a full recovery might not have especially strong feelings about the experience, while someone returning from a prolonged or unexpected hospital stay may feel that her life has been profoundly changed by the experience. Some of the psychological reactions common in recently discharged patients include:

Relief

If your loved one was seriously ill or injured but is now on the road to recovery, she may feel a great sense of relief and gratitude that things did not turn out far worse. Your best response is to listen to your loved one and share your own sense of gratitude that she is healing and recovering. If your loved one seems to be expecting too much too soon, you might try a gentle reminder to keep expectations realistic, such as, "I know the doctor said you would be 'good as new', but it might be a little soon to return to all of your pre-hospitalization activities just yet." In most cases, however, the best response is support and validation of your loved one's positive outlook.

Increased Sense of Spirituality

An increased sense of spirituality is especially common if the patient realizes he or she came very close to death, also called a "near-death experience", or is suffering from a terminal illness. Most times, renewed spirituality is a healthy, life-affirming sign, but if your loved one is using religion as a way to beat up on herself ("God's punishing me because I drank that night."), utilize support in the form of clergy at her religious center or the pastoral care services at the hospital. If she is on hospice, a chaplain will make regular visits to help you and your loved one work through any spiritual issues and, ideally, find a sense of peace and meaning.

Frustration

We live in a fast-paced world. Brief, solution-focused therapy is the name of the game. Problems get sorted out in less than an hour on television shows. Even our food usually takes five minutes or less to prepare in the microwave. It's little wonder, then, that if your loved one was seriously ill or injured, she may be frustrated with the amount of time her recovery is taking. A great response to frustration is empathy. Don't try to talk your loved one out of what she is feeling—it won't work, and it is likely to add to her sense of frustration. Instead, a better approach may be offering a statement of understanding such as, "Mom, I know you'd rather be out golfing. It must be very difficult to be stuck in the house all day when you're used to being so active."

You might also have a word with your loved one's physician or physical therapist to see if they can provide your loved one with a more realistic timeframe for recovery.

Anger

Anger is a natural reaction when forced to make significant life changes, but, as anger is frequently misplaced and projected on nearby targets, it can be a very trying emotion for the caregiver to handle.

Todd, for instance, was diagnosed with Type I diabetes when he was ten years old. His early years were marked by neglect of his condition, and most of the time, Todd didn't follow a diabetic diet, check his blood-glucose levels or take his insulin injections. As a result, Todd developed complications and had to have both legs amputated above the knee. Now confined to a wheelchair, he again refused to take any responsibility for regulating his diabetes. More infections and amputations followed, and by the time Todd was 25, he was in dire health straights.

He was also furious. When family and friends came to visit him, he cursed at them and turned to face the wall until they went away. When mental health professionals and chaplains came into his room to talk, he hurled everything he could get his hands on at them until they retreated. He was rude to his doctors and nurses. Todd had every right to be angry. Angry at his illness, angry at his mother who never took the time to teach him to control it and angry at himself for not taking better care of himself as an adult. The problem was, he displaced his anger. Everyone and everything became the enemy and he made himself and everyone around him miserable.

If your loved one is angry, you need to find the difficult balance between accepting the anger as a normal emotion and not allowing yourself to be abused. Sometimes, you may be able to assist your loved one by helping her name her anger and its target. ("You're right. It's not fair that you have this disease. I'd be angry, too.") Another helpful technique is to help your loved one find a safe way to express her anger such as hitting a pillow, scribbling in a notebook or channeling the rage into physical therapy exercises.

Caroline, who died of lung disease in her 70's, had a unique way of dealing with her anger. She would go to a thrift shop and buy the prettiest glass dishes she could find. When she returned home, she smashed every piece of that glass on her cement patio. Then she carefully swept up the shards and used them to create beautiful collages which her friends still treasure, even ten years after her death.

One way of expressing anger that is not acceptable is being emotionally or physically abusive to you or to anyone else. If your loved one is cognitively intact and calls you names, throws things, or tries to hit or kick you, impose the adult version of a "time out." Simply say something like, "Amy, I can't deal with you when you yell at me or strike out at me, so I'm going to take a walk. I'll be back in about half an hour and we can try to talk about it again."

(Note: Never go off and leave your loved one in an unsafe setting.)

Anxiety

Anxiety is a hallmark of certain disorders, especially the disorders that involve difficulty breathing, such as chronic obstructive pulmonary disease (COPD) or congestive heart failure (CHF).

People who are very anxious tend to become clingy and manipulative, two traits that do not often inspire compassion in caregivers.

One woman, for instance, whenever her daughter would need to leave, would sigh dramatically and say, "I'll probably be dead when you get back." The daughter felt like she could not have a life of her own and she resented that fact and came to resent her mother as well. When hospice workers came out to see the patient, they helped explain to the daughter that the anxiety her mother experienced was a natural result of the disease. They made sure the woman had plenty of back-up oxygen tanks and knew how to use them. They also arranged for her to get a personal alarm so, in the event of an emergency, she could call for help with the push of a button. One afternoon a week, a hospice volunteer came out to stay with the woman while her daughter ran errands or took a much-needed break. These interventions relieved the woman's anxiety enough that she was able to cut back on using manipulative techniques to keep her daughter by her side at all times.

If your loved one is experiencing a lot of anxiety be as kind and supportive as possible. Look for ways to ease the anxiety where you can, but do not allow your life to be completely controlled by your loved one's irrational fears.

It's important that you don't try to talk your loved one out of her fears; they are very real to her. Instead, simply acknowledge that it is not realistic for you to take care of all of your loved one's fears and needs and explore other options. Perhaps your loved one would be more comfortable hiring a live-in caregiver so that someone is available around the clock, or perhaps, as in the case of the woman above, your loved one simply wants to be able to contact help in the event of an emergency.

Moodiness

Most people who are making a long recuperation from an illness or injury experience fluctuations in mood. On good days, they may feel as if their therapy and medication are helping and that they are only a breath away from getting back to their old selves. On bad days, they may feel worse and fear that things may never return to the way they were before the illness or injury occurred.

Your best bet for dealing with moodiness is to be calm and realistic as your loved one recuperates. You don't want to personify "Pollyanna," forcing a silver lining to every situation, but you don't want to turn into a "Debby Downer," either. For instance, if your loved one is in pain and experiencing a bad mood, you might say something validating and practical, along the lines of, "The physical therapist warned us you'd have good days and bad days. I'm sorry this is one of the bad ones. Let me get you something to help the pain."

Sadness

Sadness is distinct from depression, which we'll examine later in the chapter. Sadness usually involves feelings of regret or mourning over one or two aspects of one's life. For instance, if your loved one has been diagnosed with a terminal illness, sadness that life is coming to an end is certainly a normal response. By the same token, if your loved one was involved in a car crash that killed a close friend, it is normal for her to feel grief after that loss.

Our instinct is often to try to "cheer up" someone who is feeling sad, but this approach is usually not successful and met with resistance. The person experiencing sadness is likely to think you simply don't understand. She may stop talking about the sadness to you, but this doesn't mean that the sadness has disappeared.

The best approach is to provide empathy and active listening as your loved one sorts through her emotions. It may even help your loved one feel understood and validated if you express some of your own sadness. ("I hate it that this is happening to you. It breaks my heart.")

Depression

Sadness usually involves one or two areas of a person's life. For instance, they're sad because their friend has died, but they can still enjoy interacting with other friends, getting back into their old routines and doing the things that previously brought them pleasure.

Depression, on the other hand, is an overwhelming condition that overcomes almost every aspect of your loved one's life. Symptoms of depression include a pervasive sense of sadness or emptiness that lasts for at least a few weeks and interferes in the daily life of your loved one. People who are depressed often feel guilty, worthless, or ashamed. They may eat too much, or not enough. They may want to stay in bed all day, or they may be unable to sleep at all. They lose interest in activities that were once enjoyable. Some people who are depressed have problems concentrating, remembering and making decisions. In fact, depression is frequently mistaken for dementia in older patients.

Major depression is a mental illness. Your loved one can't "snap out of it" any more than she could snap out of having diabetes or heart disease. If you see signs of major depression in your loved one, it's important to help her arrange to see a doctor or psychotherapist as soon as possible. Depression is very often treatable through medication or therapy. There's no reason why your loved one can't recover from it and go on to live a productive, fulfilling life.

A Word about Suicide

When you listen to news reports, you hear a lot of talk about teen suicide. While that is certainly a problem that needs to be addressed, the reports leave out the fact that the demographic most at risk group for suicide is a white male over the age of 65. Women attempt suicide more often than men, but men complete the act more often because they are more likely to use highly lethal methods like a gun.

If you suspect your loved one is considering suicide, talk to him about it and allow him the opportunity to express his feelings verbally so that he doesn't have to act them out physically.

When you bring up the issue of suicide, be compassionate but direct: "Have you had any thoughts of hurting or killing yourself?" If your loved one answers yes, assess further. Does he have a plan? Does he have the means to carry out the plan? Does he know when he would act on the plan?

Someone who simply thinks, "It would be better if I weren't here," but has no plan and no way to commit suicide is a fairly low risk. If, on the other hand, your loved one has a plan ("I'd shoot myself with the gun in the garage while you were at work and the kids were at school."), his risk is much higher. In the aforementioned example, any means to commit suicide should be removed from the home and a doctor should be contacted immediately. Regardless of how extreme the sentiment is, suicide is a very serious matter that should be dealt with by professionals.

Resource Corner: If your loved one has expressed suicidal thoughts or behavior, you can help by placing a call to a suicide preventing hotline or a local crisis center. These can be found with a simple online search.

A Word about Mental Illness

If your loved one suffers from a major mental illness like chronic depression, bipolar disorder (formerly known as manic-depressive disorder), schizophrenia or a personality disorder, don't be surprised if they have an acute episode after being discharged from hospital. Simply being in a hospital setting is upsetting even for people who do not have a mental illness. For those who do, it can easily make their symptoms worse.

Another factor that can contribute to worsening symptoms or the onset of an episode is that if your loved one has been in the hospital for a health problem, the doctors may not have made her psychiatric medications a priority, so she may come out of the hospital with her regimen of psychiatric medications altered or altogether abandoned.

Being in the hospital also disrupts sleep cycle, exercise routines, diet and other lifestyle measures your loved one may use to keep his or her symptoms under control.

There are two steps that can reduce the risk of major problems arising. First, as soon as your loved one goes into the hospital, notify her psychiatrist. The psychiatrist can talk to colleagues on staff at the hospital and make sure your loved one is observed and treated for any disturbing symptoms.

The second thing that you can do is encourage your loved one to make an appointment to see a psychiatrist as soon as she gets out of the hospital. The psychiatrist can look over the list of medications with which your loved one was discharged and make sure the medications that keep the psychiatric disorder under control have not been forgotten.

Finally, if your loved one sees a psychologist, help her get back in touch with the same professional after a hospitalization. The therapist may be able to help your loved one develop coping strategies to use in conjunction with her medication.

This chapter explored some of the major emotional/psychological issues your loved one may deal with after a hospitalization. The next chapter looks at mobility, exercise and ways that your loved one can get back on her feet as quickly as possible.

CHAPTER EIGHT
Post-Discharge Concerns: Mobility/Exercise

Years ago, doctors encouraged people who had been hospitalized for an illness or injury to stay in bed for long periods of "recuperation." Today, this is no longer the standard recommendation. In fact, patients who are able to get up and move around have better outcomes than patients who are confined to a bed.

Exactly how much activity is allowed or encouraged varies from patient to patient. Always speak to your loved one's physician or physical therapist before initiating or stepping up an exercise program.

Benefits of Exercise/Mobility

As long as a patient's doctor agrees, he or she will receive several benefits from physical activity.

Studies show that exercising for 30 minutes a day, three to five times a week, can improve mood in depressed patients. In fact, exercise can be just as effective as antidepressants or psychotherapy in improving depression symptoms.

Getting up and around will also help enhance feelings of self-sufficiency. This is especially true if the individual lives alone—or lived alone prior to the hospitalization—or has a history of enjoying sports and physical activities such as hiking, hunting, fishing, or jogging.

Another benefit of mobility and exercise is that it reduces recently discharged patients' risk of medical complications such as blood clots or pneumonia.

Finally, the sooner your loved one is able to get up and around, the greater the chance that he will regain or even surpass his prior level of mobility.

Assigned Exercises/Activities

Because the health benefits of mobility are so evident, many patients are sent home from the hospital with assigned exercises or activities. These can be as vague as an instruction to "walk as tolerated" to as specific as a list of exercises that must be performed several times every day. These exercises are usually intended to stretch and strengthen the muscles and to encourage people to resume their normal daily activities. For instance when Jack, the patient with the broken hip, returned home from his rehabilitation program, he was given 30 minutes of stretching and strengthening exercises to do every morning and every evening.

Some patients are enthusiastic about these exercise regimens, viewing them as a way to regain mobility and independence as soon as possible. Other patients, however, are less cooperative. The recommended exercises may be uncomfortable, time-consuming, or even painful.

If your loved one is not diligent in his prescribed exercise program, talk to him in order to understand what factors are keeping him from following the regimen. Encourage him to brainstorm with you to resolve the issue. For instance, if your loved one finds the exercises boring and time-consuming, perhaps he could do them while watching the news or another favorite television program. Since exercise is also beneficial for the caregiver, a good solution is to have the caregiver and discharged patient act as "exercise buddies" who encourage and motivate each other.

Many people give up on assigned exercise programs in just a few days because they don't recognize an immediate improvement in strength or mobility. Explain to your loved one that it may take several weeks before he sees concrete evidence that the exercises are paying off and helping him get better. Doctors may also prescribe exercises and activities to maintain a patient's current level of functioning. If this is the case, tell your loved one that the exercises have been assigned to keep his condition from getting worse. Emphasize that if he stops the exercises, he may lose the mobility he currently has.

If pain is the issue, speak with the doctor or physical therapist. The doctor may prescribe a different pain medication or advise using current pain medications half an hour before the individual is ready to begin exercising.

If your loved one refuses to comply with a prescribed exercise regimen, notify the doctor or the physical therapist who prescribed it. The treatment team may be able to suggest an exercise or activity that your loved one finds more appealing. At the very least, they will be aware of the situation as they continue to coordinate your loved one's care.

Too Much Exercise?

At the opposite end of the non-compliance spectrum is the patient who tries to do too much too soon. When Andrea, 56, had a complete hysterectomy, for instance, her doctor advised her to avoid housework and heavy lifting. When she was released from the hospital, Andrea returned to her home where she lived alone and went right back to her routine of vacuuming, doing frequent loads of laundry and lifting heavy cartons of the cat litter.

Andrea's over-activity caused her surgical wound to re-open and become infected. She had to go back to the hospital where she received wound care and IV antibiotics. When she was ready to return home again, her doctor arranged for a home health nurse to continue the wound care. Andrea also hired a private-duty home care agency to assist with tasks like light housekeeping and meal preparation. Her next door neighbor agreed to help with caring for the cats.

Because of all the support in place, Andrea's second homecoming was much more successful than her first. She eventually went on to make a full recovery.

If your loved one is engaging in an activity you believe to be unsafe, notify his doctor. If the doctor agrees that the activity is not a good idea, ask the doctor to talk with your loved one. He might be more likely to listen to a physician than to you.

If any activity—even one that the doctor has prescribed—causes a recently discharged patient to experience intense pain, bleeding, dizziness, or extreme shortness of breath, the activity should be stopped immediately and a doctor should be consulted.

Illness versus Surgery

Research suggests that older clients with an illness such as chronic obstructive pulmonary disease (COPD) or congestive heart failure (CHF) are more likely to decline physically after a hospitalization than elderly patients who were injured or underwent surgery. Patients with non-surgical illnesses also tended to be more depressed than their counterparts who required surgery.

Although these statistics may seem puzzling at first, they make sense when you consider that surgical patients are more likely to be referred for rehabilitation and given an exercise regimen to perform at home. In other words, the medical staff expects their conditions to improve and treats them accordingly.

Of course, patients with chronic or terminal illnesses are not expected to improve. Rather than recommending exercises to promote mobility, doctors often tell these patients to limit their physical activity. These patients may feel hopeless and sink into a depression which leads to both physical and cognitive declines.

If your loved one has returned from the hospital after an illness, emphasize what he can do rather than what he can't. For instance, if the doctor has ordered continuous oxygen, ask the medical equipment company to provide a portable oxygen system and take your loved one on short walks around the neighborhood. You can also promote healthy activity by encouraging your loved one to participate in his or her own care as much as possible.

Keeping recently discharged patients as active as the medical team will allow boosts their mental and physical wellbeing. The next chapter will describe the ways that proper nutrition also plays a role in the care of a patient after hospitalization.

CHAPTER NINE
Post-Discharge Concerns: Nutrition

Obesity is a growing health concern across the United States and Canada. Studies place the obesity rate between 20% and 30% in both these countries. There are several reasons for this dangerous trend:

- People's jobs require much more sitting and much less exercise.

- Delicious, high-calorie foods are available at every drive-through restaurant.

- Many people are emotional eaters, using food to comfort themselves.

- People who live alone may not want to go to the trouble of preparing a healthy meal and instead just eat "whatever is in the fridge."

Worse, since people tend to gravitate towards comfort foods – chocolate, ice cream, potato chips, starches, etc. – most of the calories they eat are "empty calories," or calories that contain no vitamins, proteins, irons, or other nutrients. What many people outside the medical profession don't understand is that it's possible, and quite common, to be simultaneously obese and malnourished.

Donna, for instance, was 60 years old and weighed nearly 300 pounds when her adult son, Max, brought her to the hospital emergency room after noting that she was more tired than usual and seemed to be getting increasingly forgetful. Max knew there was a history of Alzheimer's in the family and he feared his mother was showing the first symptoms. Instead, blood tests revealed malnourishment. Donna admitted she'd been depressed and hadn't had anything but chocolate to eat and soda to drink for the last three weeks.

She was discharged home with orders to follow a strict diet and exercise program and a referral to a therapist to get a handle on her depression and her problems with food. After a few weeks of following her new regimen, Donna had lost a dozen pounds and her depression, fatigue, and forgetfulness had all improved. Blood tests further corroborated the progress in her health status.

In the Hospital

When a person is hospitalized, the family often approaches the doctor to express concerns about whether or not the individual has been eating properly. If you have those concerns, you may ask the doctor to order a nutritional consult. A nutritionist talks to the patient, her family and the medical staff and gathers other information such as lab test results. Based on his or her findings, the nutritionist may recommend dietary changes. While providing education about the body's need for certain types of fuel (food), the nutritionist will generally work with a patient to come up with a diet with which he or she can live.

After all, the most brilliant diet plan in the world won't work if your loved one won't follow it. That is why it is important that she play a role in choosing the foods she wants to eat with the guidance of a nutritionist to fulfill her nutritional requirements.

If a person is on a special diet or has been hospitalized for a nutrition-related issue, it is important to bring only healthy foods – or no foods at all – to the hospital. Debra Stang, a medical social worker, vividly remembers cases where family members would express shock and horror that a patient's diabetes was so poorly managed or that she was malnourished. Almost invariably when Stang dropped by the patient's room to go over discharge plans, the floor would be strewn with wrappers from candy bars or other "forbidden" treats. If your loved one is putting pressure on you to help her cheat, refuse gently but firmly.

("Sorry, Mom, but the doctor says no," or "Right now you're on a pretty strict diet. Maybe you can have some ice cream another time.")

It's also a good idea to let other family members and friends who visit your loved one know about her new diet plan as well. Again, you can be firm, but tactful ("It's so nice of you to offer to bring Mom fudge, and I'm sure she'd enjoy it, but the doctors are being pretty strict with what she eats right now and I want to try to support their decision.")

Community Resources

Older people often start having nutritional issues after a spouse has died. They don't like to cook for themselves anymore and frozen dinners, while easy to prepare, are usually not healthy. Sometimes, financial problems will keep a patient from eating as she should. Stang states that several patients have revealed to her that, with pharmaceutical costs skyrocketing, they feel as if they have to choose between buying their medicine and buying nutritious food.

There are a number of nutritional resources available to seniors. Most communities offer a home delivered meals program (e.g. Meals on Wheels), often through a local council or agency on aging. Home delivered meal programs usually request a donation, but they will not stop services if the patient cannot afford them. Home delivered meals provide 1/3 of the nutrients required in a day. Most programs are not able to prepare special meals for people who must eat low cholesterol, low sodium, or diabetic diets.

Most communities also have one or more "senior centers," often affiliated with the local community or recreation center. These are places where older adults can go to socialize, play games, enjoy entertainment and eat a nutritious meal. If your loved one has talked to you about feeling lonely and is still able to leave the home without assistance, encourage her to go to the local senior center for lunch or dinnertime.

Post-Discharge

Ask your loved one's doctor or nutritionist if she or he needs to follow a special diet. Diabetics, for instance, are usually warned not to eat too much sugar and people with heart disease may require a low-sodium diet. If a person has a surgical wound that is healing, the doctor may encourage her to eat extra protein to promote faster healing and recuperation.

If the absence of other instructions, according to the Department of Agriculture in their 2010 Dietary Guidelines, the average woman between the ages of 31 and 50 requires 1,800 calories per day to maintain her weight. A woman over the age of 50 needs only 1,600 calories to maintain her weight. Men who are age 31 to 50, on the other hand, require 2,200 calories to maintain their weight. Even men over the age of 51 should eat at least 2,000 calories per day to maintain energy and blood sugar levels.

About half of these calories should come from fruits and vegetables. Other healthy options to round out your loved one's diet include fat-free and low-fat dairy products such as milk and cheese, whole grains, poultry, seafood and unsalted mixed nuts for protein.

Another positive nutrition habit for discharged patients to develop is to substitute water for drinks with sugar and caffeine such as soda and coffee.

Of course, you will have to work with your loved one to initiate these dietary changes if they are not already in practice. If you suddenly start serving food that is outside of a person's comfort zone, they may initially resist and refuse to eat it. It may take a few tries to find a healthy comprises that satisfy both your loved ones palate and health. A great first step is sitting down together to create a sample menu for the day and working from that.

Special Treats

There's an old joke about a man who goes to his doctor and says, "I've done everything you asked. I've given up sweets. I threw away my cigarettes. I haven't had a drink in six months. I jog twice a day, I drive the speed limit and wear my seatbelt. I gave up my girlfriend. Now remind me again why I am doing all these things."

"So you can live longer, of course!" the doctor exclaims. The man eyes him bleakly for a minute and says, "Why?"

There is a kernel of truth in this joke. The focus is not only length of life, but also quality of life. And for many individuals, indulging in the occasional treat adds to their quality of life. Your loved one should maintain a healthy diet as much as possible but that shouldn't preclude the possibility of occasional treats like sharing ice cream cones with a grandchild or enjoying a second helping at Thanksgiving dinner. The important thing is not to slip into making every day a "special treat" day.

Nutritional Supplements

Many individuals coming home following a hospital stay report a dramatic reduction in appetite. They may still feel physically unwell, which is an appetite suppressant. Some are struggling with depression or anxiety, which can also decrease the appetite. The relationship between appetite, physical activity and food leads to a vicious cycle where an individual doesn't feel well which impacts her appetite, not eating makes her weaker and too tired to engage in any physical activity, the lack of physical activity coupled with not eating makes her feel worse, and so on.

If you're struggling to get your loved one to consume necessary calories, ask your doctor about a nutritional supplement such as Boost, Ensure or Glucerna (for diabetics). Nutritional supplements only take a few minutes to drink and they will deliver the much-needed calories and nutrients.

Nutritional supplements come in many different flavors, and while very few people would pick them as a "favorite food," most are able to find a flavor that they enjoy most. Try buying one of each flavor and allowing your loved one to pick a favorite before investing in a larger package. Nutritional supplements taste best when they are very cold. If your loved one can't (or doesn't want to) drink a whole bottle, pour a small amount into a paper cup and ask her to drink it. Put the rest of the bottle back into the refrigerator. Periodically throughout the day, pour a little more of the supplement into the cup and encourage your loved one to "just take a sip." The goal is for her to have finished the bottle by the end of the day.

Another way to help your loved one get the vitamins she needs is to start giving her a multivitamin every day. If she complains that the vitamin is too large to swallow, you can try cutting it into pieces or crushing it and mixing it with applesauce, Jell-O, or a small dish of ice cream.

Hospice

If your loved one is on hospice, the goal is to maintain and enhance her quality of life as much as possible for as long as she has left to live (usually six months or fewer). At this point, doctors focus less on emphasizing that patients stick to a certain diet and care more about ensuring the person is comfortable. You start hearing phrases like, "All calories are good calories." Shortly before the end of life, many people slip into a brief coma and stop eating and drinking completely. This can be frightening for family members who assume their loved ones are "starving to death," but it is just a normal part of the dying process. The body is no longer able to handle food. If a terminally ill patient starts losing interest in food, remind yourself as often as necessary that diminished appetite is a natural part of the dying process.

This chapter provided guidance in helping the post-hospital patient maintain proper nutrition. The next chapter will look at hygiene, personal care and the types of assistance a discharged patient might need to feel and look his or her best.

CHAPTER TEN
Post-Discharge Concerns:
Hygiene, Personal Care and Fall Prevention

Hygiene and personal care consists of the routine your loved one follows to look and feel his or her best. The most common types of personal care include:

- Getting up and getting dressed in the morning and getting ready for bed at night
- Brushing teeth (2-3 times per day)
- Shaving
- Applying makeup
- Keeping hands clean throughout the day
- Going to the bathroom or putting on/changing briefs/ adult diapers
- Showering or bathing (3 times per week)

Caring for fingernails and toenails as needed (if your loved one is diabetic, let a podiatrist handle the toenail care)

Before your loved one leaves the hospital, talk to the nursing staff or the physical therapy staff to get an idea of his level of independence with personal care. If you don't think you can manage your loved one's care by yourself, speak up before he is discharged from the hospital. Ask to speak to the social worker or the discharge planner. They can help you plan for additional care in the home, most commonly provided by non-medical caregivers. For patients who require additional support or who lack a safe home environment, a nursing facility or rehabilitation center may be a good alternative to explore.

Preparing the Bathroom

The bathroom is the room in the house where people handle most of their physical care. If your loved one is still relatively independent, you can help him by making sure the bathroom is as user-friendly as possible.

Some suggestions for enhancing your bathroom include placing grab bars inside the tub or the shower and on the wall next to the toilet. A discharged patient should never use the towel rack to pull himself up or to support his weight. The towel rack is not installed to bear the weight of a person and it may pull away from the wall, causing your loved one to lose his balance and fall. Grab bars, on the other hand, are designed specifically to withstand a certain amount of weight and pressure, and individuals can safely rely on them.

Getting up and down from a low toilet seat can be difficult for someone who is weak or who suffers from joint pain due to arthritis. It may help to purchase a toilet riser. A toilet riser is like a bedside commode without the bucket to catch waste material. It goes over the toilet, providing individuals a seat several inches higher than the average toilet. If your loved one has trouble making it to the bathroom on time, you may also want to purchase a plastic urinal or hand-held plastic container used to catch urine. A urinal can be used in any room in the house.

Once you are satisfied that your loved one will be safe using the toilet, turn your attention to bathing and showering. A non-slip mat in and beside the tub may make the process of getting clean easier and less anxiety-provoking for your loved one. Even people who are in the best of health sometimes slip and fall on slick floors, and if a person is unsteady on his feet, his chances of a fall are significantly increased.

Another thing you can do to make the bathroom safer is to purchase a tub bench. A tub bench is a bench about the height of an average chair. It enables individuals to sit down while showering. Even if your loved one is sure that he is strong enough to shower standing up, it doesn't hurt to have the bench available in case of emergencies. People who are discharged from the hospital after a significant illness or injury are often weaker than they realize. Having a tub bench in place allows an individual the freedom to shower while standing if he pleases, while giving him a safe place to rest if he becomes tired or loses strength in his legs.

If your loved one lives alone or if you live in a large house where you might not be able to hear a call for help, renting a personal medical alarm is a good idea. A personal medical alarm such as Lifeline or Life Alert allows your loved one to call for help by touching a call button worn on a durable bracelet or necklace. Some alarm systems are so sophisticated that they can actually detect a fall even if the individual is not alert enough to press the button to summon help. The alarm jewelry is waterproof, so one can wear it even while showering or bathing.

Some people are resistant to the idea of using personal alarms at first. One patient complained that he felt like he was "on a leash." It may help to explain to your loved one that the alarm actually gives him more independence because it makes you feel better about him living on his own.

Levels of Assistance

Before your loved one returns home from the hospital, ask the hospital staff to assess how well he manages the activities involved in personal care, also called the activities of daily living or ADLs.

If your loved one is independent, it means he can safely be left alone to provide care for himself.

If you loved one requires stand-by assistance, you or a caregiver need to be present to provide physical assistance and coaching as necessary. Always allow the patient to do as much as possible for himself, but be ready to lend a helping hand if he can't step out of the tub on his own or if he needs someone to help him tie his shoes.

If individual has cognitive impairments because of Alzheimer's disease or another type of dementia, he may be able to physically handle the tasks of self-care, but you or a caregiver may need to gently coach him and make suggestions if he forgets what he is doing. When cueing your loved one, use short sentences and offer one idea at a time. For instance, if you say, "Stand up, wipe yourself off, pull up your pants, and do up the zipper," your loved one is likely to forget most of what you have said which can lead to both of you becoming frustrated and discouraged. Instead, wait until your loved one completes one task before cueing him for the next.

You may also need to provide light physical guidance. If you are telling him, for example, to put his right arm through the sleeve, lightly touch his right hand or gently guide his arm into the proper position.

Many people who are just getting out of the hospital after an illness or injury have good days and bad days. On their bad days, they may need a lot of physical assistance to complete the activities of daily living. On their good days, they may be close to independent. Since your loved one may not always be able to tell you that he is having a bad day, watch for behavioral indicators like confusion, stumbling, or skipping personal care tasks because he is unable to perform them. Be ready to provide as much help as needed.

If your loved one is confined to a bed or a wheelchair, he may need extensive or complete physical assistance. This means that you or a caregiver will be primarily responsible for cleaning and grooming him. This may be difficult and awkward in any situation, but it is an especially touchy area for adult children taking care of their parents.

If you find yourself physically or emotionally unable to provide the care your loved one needs, you can make arrangements for someone else to help. Some people are able to find a family member, friend, or neighbor who is willing to lend a hand, but most people in this situation choose to hire a caregiver from a private duty care agency. Caregivers are trained to provide assistance to patients in all of their daily activities, and many adult children report that having a caregiver allows them to maintain and grow the quality of their relationship with their parent. Another option is arranging for your loved one to go to a nursing facility where the staff will be able to care for him.

Privacy

As mentioned in the previous section, providing personal care to a loved one can be awkward at first. The best way to put your loved one at ease is to preserve his privacy as much as possible. You can do this in several ways.

First, encourage your loved one to be as independent as possible. This can be frustrating for caregivers who know that their loved one will take over an hour to get dressed on his own while they could dress him in ten minutes. Having the individual do things for himself, though, can raise self-esteem, help alleviate depression and sometimes spare you from having to provide intimate care that can make your loved one feel uncomfortable.

If you need to bathe the individual or provide perennial care (care around the genitals and rectum), approach him in a matter-of-fact, calm manner and explain exactly what you are going to do before you do it.

When you bathe your loved one, only uncover the part of the body you're working on at that time. For instance, if you are bathing the right arm, his chest, left arm, genitals and legs should be covered.

Caregiver Safety

Many caregivers, even professional caregivers, who are required to provide heavy physical assistance to their patients, end up straining or spraining their backs. These tips can help keep you injury-free.

- When lifting something heavy, squat and lift with the power of your legs. Do not stoop over and use the muscles of your back to lift.

- Raise the bed to a comfortable level when providing care so you don't have to bend over. Remember to lower the bed again when the task is complete.

- Use a gait belt to help the patient transfer from one place to another.

- Ask the doctor about getting a mechanical lift for transfers.

- Hire assistance if you need to.

Remember, you don't have to be a hero and do everything alone. Keep the lines of communication open with your family, and if you need extra help, ask for it. Otherwise, you are at risk of becoming ill or injured yourself.

Falls

When you are helping with your loved one's personal care, you may have to deal with a fall. Some falls occur because of slips and trips, but many happen because the individual simply loses strength in his legs. Another cause of falling is missing the edge of the chair while trying to sit down. Individuals, especially older adults, may also suffer a "pathological fracture." This occurs when a bone in the leg or hip breaks due to osteoporosis or another disease process. The fracture causes individuals to lose their balance and fall.

If your loved one starts to fall, don't try to catch him or prevent the fall. Instead, use the gait belt or the waistband of the pants to lower him to the floor as gently as possible.

Once he is on the floor, assess him for injury. Make sure he is not in pain and can move his arms and legs. Call an ambulance if you suspect a broken bone or if the individual has hit his head during the fall.

If you are convinced that he is not injured, see if he can get back on his feet. If he is able to get his legs under him and push against the floor with his feet, you may be able to use his gait belt to help him back to a standing position. Whatever you do, do not stoop over and pull on your loved one's arms. This puts both of you at risk for injury.

It isn't easy to help someone off the floor by yourself. You may need to summon a neighbor or another family member to help out. If there is no one you can call, dial 911 and tell them your loved one needs help after a "non-emergency fall."

Emphasize that your loved one is not injured and does not require transportation to the hospital, only assistance getting off the floor.

If your loved one can't get off the floor, stay with him until help arrives. Make him as comfortable as possible by covering him with a blanket and placing a pillow under his head. Hold his hand and reassure him that everything will be all right.

It is not unusual for people to be at increased risk of falls following a hospitalization. Do not blame yourself if your loved one has a fall in your care. Simply continue to provide comfort and companionship until help arrives.

The last few chapters have provided advice on how to handle common issues that may come up in a patient's care after a hospitalization. The next several chapters will look at common reasons why people are hospitalized and their unique needs after being discharged. The first chapter will deal with acute, or sudden onset, medical problems that can lead to a hospital stay

CHAPTER ELEVEN
Acute Medical Problems

Acute medical problems are medical problems that have a sudden onset. This chapter discusses four common reasons why individuals undergo unexpected hospitalizations and how you can help them continue to improve upon their return home.

Pneumonia

Pneumonia is far more treatable now than it was even a few decades ago. Pneumonia is a bacterial, viral, or fungal infection in one or both lungs. The infection causes the lungs to become inflamed and the person with pneumonia may complain of chest pain or trouble breathing. The most common treatments for pneumonia include antibiotics and rest.

While younger patients may be sent home to recuperate, older adults, people who smoke on a regular basis, people whose immune systems are compromised, and people with certain lung ailments are especially vulnerable to developing complications. If your loved one fits into one or more of these categories, she will probably be admitted for observation and treatment with intravenous (IV) antibiotics. Your loved one's doctor may do a lung biopsy or a culture their sputum to determine what type of pneumonia they have and whether or not it is antibiotic resistant.

Pneumonia can cause several life-threatening complications in vulnerable patients. One of the most dreaded complications is sepsis, which occurs when the infection travels from the lungs into the bloodstream. Once there, it is circulated throughout the body where it may attack other organs, causing multi-organ failure. Another complication is Adult Respiratory Distress Syndrome or ARDS. Even after years of research, the causes of ARDS remain unclear, and the survival rate is still around 50%. Finally, the infection inside the lungs may cause infected fluid to build up outside of the lungs as well, making breathing painful and difficult.

Home Care Considerations: Your loved one will probably be given oral antibiotics to take for several days after she returns home from the hospital. If the physician believes that IV drugs would be more effective, he or she can work with the discharge planner to arrange for a home health agency to manage the IVs.

If a person's lungs have been damaged by the infection, she may need to be on oxygen for a period of time. Medicare pays 80% of the cost for medical equipment such as oxygen concentrators and emergency oxygen tanks. If you have a Medicare supplement plan, it will probably cover the remaining 20% of the charges. Again, your discharge planner can help you find a company that will take your insurance. The discharge planner will also order the equipment for you.

Follow the doctor's instructions about when the oxygen should be used. The doctor may order it for nights only, prn (as needed) or continuous use. Individuals wearing oxygen should not smoke, light candles, or go near any other source of flame. If a person on oxygen insists on smoking, take the oxygen tubing off her face, shut off the concentrator and move it to another room while the individual has her cigarette.

Before leaving the hospital, be sure you understand how active the discharged patient can be. Until she gets her strength back, the medical staff is likely to suggest brief periods of non-impact activities such as walking followed by periods of rest.

Pneumonia is an illness that may reoccur just when you thought the person was improving. If your loved one develops a high fever (in the elderly, this may translate into a lower than normal temperature), cough or chest pain, bring her back to the doctor for immediate evaluation.

Emotional Considerations. An individual's emotions may vary widely after coming home from the hospital. A person may be traumatized by the sudden onset of the illness, relieved that she survived or upset because she now needs to be on oxygen. Additionally, people who have trouble catching their breath may become anxious and fearful, often to the point of becoming extraordinarily clingy to those around them.

You can best support your loved one by listening to her concerns. You don't have to find solutions or make promises that can't be kept ("You'll be good as new in a couple of days!"), but if her take on the future seems overly pessimistic, you can inject a little reality by saying something like, "I didn't hear the doctor say that. I thought he said…"

A recently discharged patient one may also have spiritual and legal concerns after facing a scary, life-threatening illness. You can help by arranging for her to get in touch with a member of the clergy at her church or by calling an attorney that specializes in legal matters that affect the elderly.

Shingles

Shingles is a painful rash caused by varicella-zoster virus, the same virus that causes chicken pox. When we have chicken pox as kids, the virus never leaves our body. Instead, it lies inactive near the brain and spinal cord or the central nervous system. If the virus becomes active again, for reasons that are not fully understood, the result is shingles.

Shingles usually occur in small patches on one side of the chest or stomach. The first symptom is usually pain, tingling, or numbness in the area. A few days later, a rash appears on the skin. The rash contains fluid-filled blisters that open, weep, and then crust over. As the rash starts to heal, the person with shingles may complain of itching.

The people most vulnerable to shingles are those over the age of 65 or those with an immune system weakened by a condition such as HIV/AIDS.

Shingles is not usually considered a life-threatening disease and most doctors elect to treat it outside the hospital. If your loved one is in a highly weakened state due to several other health concerns, however, her doctor might decide to admit her to the hospital for observation and pain management.

Most people make a clean recovery from shingles. The most common complication is skin infections which can enter through the open blisters. These infections can be prevented by closer attention to hygiene and treated with an antibiotic ointment. A certain percentage of recovering patients continue to experience pain in the area (postherpetic neuralgia) even after the rash has gone away and may require additional care from a pain clinic. The most serious complication, which occurs only rarely, is an inflammation of the brain called encephalitis.

Home Care Considerations. The doctor will likely send the patient home with a few medications. Most physicians opt to treat shingles with antiviral drugs. The drugs cannot cure the virus, but they can speed up the healing process and decrease the risk of complications and side effects.

Your loved one will probably have at least one and maybe even two or three medications to manage the pain. Common choices include anticonvulsants, which are effective in treating neurological pain, narcotic pain killers and topical medications that numb the skin.

Many people with shingles also find relief in cool baths or cool compresses placed on the blisters.

Individuals recovering from shingles are typically able continue with their daily routines.

The chicken pox virus can cause serious problems in newborns, pregnant women or people with significantly weakened immune systems. If your loved one shares a home with people meeting these criteria, talk to the doctor about safety precautions.

Emotional Considerations. Shingles may cause the individual a lot of pain, which may make her grumpy or difficult to be around. Remain calm and sympathetic, even if your loved one is fussy or argumentative. Use distractions to give your loved one something to think about besides her discomfort.

("Mom, will you show me how to bake and apple pie? Mine never taste as good as yours do.")

Dehydration

Dehydration is a condition which occurs when the body loses more fluids than it takes in. Dehydration may be caused by severe diarrhea or vomiting, exercising vigorously – especially in hot weather – without drinking enough fluids, or forgetting to consume fluids over a period of a day or more.

Older adults tend to be more vulnerable to severe cases of dehydration than their younger counterparts. This is because the body becomes less efficient at storing water as a person ages. Our taste buds and eating habits also change as we age, so older adults may not even be aware of feeling thirsty, a warning sign of mild dehydration. Older adults are also more likely to take laxatives or diuretics which can deplete the body of fluid. Those with cognitive impairments, such as Alzheimer's disease, may simply forget to eat or drink for a significant period of time. Older people are especially at risk during hot weather spells, especially if they don't own an air conditioner or refuse to run it for financial reasons.

Mild to moderate dehydration causes no lingering side effects and can usually be effectively treated by drinking more fluids. Severe dehydration, however, is a true medical emergency. A severely dehydrated person is at risk of death because the body cannot function without an adequate amount of fluids.

Other complications of severe dehydration include swelling of the brain (cerebral edema) during rehydration, seizures and kidney failure.

At the hospital, the patient will receive intravenous (IV) fluids. Most doctors suggest a brief admission to the hospital to find out why the dehydration occurred and to plan with the family a way to ensure that future episodes can be avoided.

Home Care Considerations. If your loved one became dehydrated during the summer months, make sure she has access to a place with air conditioning and that she is willing to use the air conditioning. Some air conditioned places to consider include libraries, movie theaters, stores and senior centers. You and other members of your family may also decide that your loved one would be better off living with one of you until the weather cools down.

It is also important to make sure that your loved one is consuming enough fluids. The best fluid of all is water, but milk, coffee, tea, juice, soda, energy drinks and even nutritional supplement shakes are all better than nothing. Many older adults experience appetite changes as they age, and may feel overwhelmed if you hand them a large glass full of liquid. Instead, offer a small glass, such as a "shot glass", full of water or juice approximately every hour.

If you work during the day and will not be around to remind your loved one to drink fluids, consider hiring a caregiver from a reputable home care agency. While providing companionship and assistance with activities of daily living, the caregiver can also encourage your loved one to take small sips of fluids regularly.

Emotional Considerations. Being rushed to the hospital after becoming dehydrated can be a traumatizing experience. Your loved one may also be traumatized by the life changes that occur afterwards, like not being able to stay alone in her apartment. Furthermore, if the dehydration incident highlighted a cognitive decline that your loved one was trying to conceal, she may be humiliated about everyone knowing she is experiencing memory loss. Allow your loved one to express her feelings of fear, frustration and even anger without judgment. Instead of trying to convince her that she has no reason to be angry, validate her feelings.

("Mom, I'd be really angry, too, if I had just gone through the same thing. But the most important thing in the world to me is keeping you safe, and I'll do what I have to do, even if it means you get upset with me sometimes.")

Bowel-Related Problems

The only bowel problem likely to warrant hospitalization is a bowel obstruction. A bowel obstruction occurs when all or part of the large or small intestine is blocked so that food, fluids, gas and feces cannot move around the obstruction. Bowel obstructions have many causes. Some of the more common ones include fecal impaction, which occurs when a person becomes so constipated that a large mass of waste gets stuck in the bowels, tumors, scar tissue, Crohn's disease and twisting of the bowel.

People with obstructions typically experience intermittent but intense cramping pains around or below the belly button. They may also vomit frequently, since the food cannot make it through the digestive system, or complain that their abdomen feels swollen or bloated. Most people with obstructions cannot pass stool. Some of the time, though, fluid feces leaks around a partial obstruction and causes diarrhea.

A bowel obstruction is almost always treated in the hospital. First a tube is placed through the nose into the patient's stomach to remove fluids and gas. The person is then given medication for pain and monitored carefully. Some obstructions simply go away on their own. Others require non-surgical interventions such as a series of enemas. If the bowel is completely blocked or if the blood supply to a part of the intestine is cut off, surgery is almost always required. (See Chapter Twelve for more information about caring for the patient recovering from surgery.)

Home Care Considerations. An individual's prognosis and follow up care are largely dependent on the cause of the obstruction. A cancerous tumor, for instance, usually means follow-up treatment with radiation or chemotherapy, while obstructions due to an impaction (severe constipation) may simply require a change in diet or medication.

In some cases, the doctor may need to operate to remove a diseased part of the colon. If so, your loved one will probably come home with a colostomy. A colostomy is created when a doctor removes part of the colon and brings the rest to the surface of the abdomen creating an opening (stoma). Fecal matter drains from the stoma into a watertight bag or pouch that is attached to the skin with adhesive. The bag needs to be emptied whenever it is one-third to one-half full. There are different types of colostomies. Before your loved one leaves the hospital, ask the nurse for specific instructions on when and how to change the colostomy bag. You might also ask for a referral to a home health agency so that a nurse can come by the house, check your loved one's colostomy and answer any questions you may have.

Complications for people with colostomies include the bowel retracting back into the abdomen, the bowel protruding too far out of the abdomen, hernias and stenosis, or narrowing of the bowel. If you suspect your loved one is having any of these complications, or if fecal material is not passing into the bag as it should, call your doctor for advice.

Emotional Considerations. Our culture typically avoids talking about the anus, rectum and bowel. You and your loved one may both be embarrassed when you talk about bowel issues. If your loved one gets a colostomy, she may be afraid to leave the home for fear of someone noticing the bag.

Try to work through your own embarrassment by talking to someone you trust or attending a support group for caregivers. Once you start talking about it, you will be surprised at how quickly the topic of bowel care becomes just another aspect of your loved one's needs. Debra Stang, a social worker and discharge planner, recalls that family members would stop by her office and say, "I can help Mom with anything but...that." With a little training and encouragement from the hospital staff, however, they soon became experts in helping their loved one with bowel-related issues.

As you become more comfortable with the topic, provide as much emotional support as you can to your parent or loved one. Handle bowel care in a calm, matter-of-fact manner. If your loved one is afraid to leave the house with her colostomy bag, remind her that the bag will be completely hidden by her clothes, and that it is watertight to prevent any leakage or unpleasant smells. Encourage her to accompany you on short outings (10 to 15 minutes) and then, as she becomes more at ease, slowly increase the time you spend out of the house.

If you find it absolutely impossible to provide bowel care, hiring a caregiver from a home care agency like Home Care Assistance to provide the care may be the best decision for you and your loved one.

This chapter examined acute medical conditions that might send your loved one to the hospital. The next chapter examines how your loved one's care may be affected by an injury or a surgery.

CHAPTER TWELVE
Accidents and Surgeries

Many people go to the hospital because they are sick, but another common cause of hospitalization among older adults is injury. The injury may be the result of a fall, or the person may suffer a pathological fracture (a fracture that occurs due to brittle bones or osteoporosis) which then causes him to fall.

Soft Tissue Injury

A soft tissue injury is a closed injury (as opposed to a cut or laceration) that does not involve the bone. Sprains, strains, contusions (bruises), tendonitis, bursitis and repetitive stress injuries are all soft tissue injuries.

In the elderly, soft tissue injuries are usually the result of a fall. In fact, according to the Journal of Epidemiology and Community Health, a fall with a soft tissue injury is a strong predictor of more serious falls and injuries to come.

Patients are usually not admitted to the hospital for a soft tissue injury. The admissions that do occur happen because the doctor wants to rule out something more serious, such as a fracture or a head injury. The doctor finds the bruises suspicious and wants to ensure the individual's safety, or they can no longer access his or her home due to the injury and the discharge planner needs time to arrange an alternative placement.

A soft tissue injury may be a sign of abuse. If you do not live with the person or were not present when the injury occurred, talk to them and to the hospital staff about how it happened. Be especially cautious about bruises that are shaped like an object (hand, fist, electric cord, etc.) or about wounds that are in unusual places. For instance, if your loved one fell forward, you might expect bruising on his hands and knees, but not on the fleshy part of his upper arm. If you suspect the person is being abused, tell the medical staff immediately and work closely with the discharge planner and the hospital social worker to make sure your loved one will be safe when he is discharged from the hospital.

Home Care Considerations. Your loved one may be stiff and sore after a fall. If he sprained an ankle, he might need crutches or a walker to get around safely. The hospital staff will help you arrange for the appropriate equipment.

The individual may experience some physical discomfort after discharge. This can usually be relieved with over the counter pain medication or a soothing bath or shower.

Emotional Considerations. If the patient suffered a fall, he may be angry and depressed. He may also be afraid of falling again and may want to stay in his bed or his chair even after the pain from the injury fades.

You can help by providing him with emotional and practical support. Allow your loved one to talk about the fall and how frightening or stressful it was. Don't discount his feelings; listen with empathy and genuine concern. On a practical level, do everything you can to prevent future falls (see Chapter Ten).

Fractures

A fracture refers to a break in an individual's bones. Of all the different types of fractures, a hip fracture is most likely to put a person out of commission for a while. According to the International Osteoporosis Foundation, there are about 1.6 million hip fractures across the globe each year; North America accounts for the majority of these fractures. Ninety percent of patients with hip fractures are over the age of 50. Hip fractures generally require surgery to repair them. The doctor and the discharge planner will probably suggest that your loved one go to a rehabilitation facility or a skilled nursing facility for extra help getting back on his feet.

Home Care Considerations. Your loved one will very likely need to use a cane, a walker, or even a wheelchair to get around. If a wheelchair is needed, make sure the doors in the home are wide enough to accommodate one. If not, the individual may need to go to a skilled nursing facility or move in with another family member until he gets back on his feet.

The most common complications of hip fractures are infections. The surgical wound may become infected if it is not kept clean. The individual may also be more vulnerable to other types of infections such as influenza or pneumonia, especially if he hasn't been getting much exercise. Call the doctor or your home health nurse immediately if your loved one's surgical wound starts to look red and puffy or if he develops other symptoms such as a bad cough and a fever.

After a hip fracture, your loved one has a 50 to 60 percent chance of regaining his previous level of mobility. His chances of having limited mobility, such as walking at home but using a wheelchair to get around in public places, are about 10 to 15 percent. About 20 percent of previously ambulatory people who fracture their hips will never walk again. It's important to realize that most the recovery will occur within six months of his injury. That is why it is so important to encourage physical therapy, even when doing so is painful. It is also important to help the individual, or enlist a caregiver, to complete any home exercises the therapist prescribes.

Emotional Considerations. As with other falls, the person may feel frightened and depressed by what has happened to him, but because hip fractures are so common, he may also feel a significant amount of hope that he will get better. Encourage hopeful thinking as much as you can. Help your loved one come up with a list of things he wants to do when his mobility improves. When one of the more difficult recovery days comes, and it will, you can say something like,

"Dad, I know it's hard, but you promised to take Mom on a cruise in June, and you won't be able to do that if you don't do your exercises."

Knee Replacement

Unlike bones in the hip, bones in the knee seldom break, but with old age and use, they can wear down, start rubbing against each other, and cause tremendous pain. If the individual is healthy enough for surgery, your doctor may suggest knee replacement.

Don't expect your loved one to be flat on his back for a long time after this surgery. The hospital staff will probably have him up and walking by the day after, if not the day of, the operation. While he is in the hospital, physical and occupational therapists will work with him on a daily basis. When he is discharged, the doctor will refer him to a home health agency that can provide therapy in the home or to a therapy center where your loved one can go for outpatient treatment.

Home Care Considerations. Your loved one will be relatively independent within a short time of the surgery, but according to the Joint Reconstruction Center at Georgetown University, he should not be alone in the house for at least four weeks post-surgery due to the risk of falls and complications. If your loved one usually lives alone, he may need to stay with you or another family member or go to a nursing facility for a few weeks until he is able to be alone again. Another option is to hire a caregiver from a private duty agency to provide care around-the-clock or on an hourly basis if the individual prefers staying at home but there are no family members or friends available to provide the companionship.

Encourage your loved one to spend as much time out of bed as possible. He should take short walks several times a day. If he insists on staying in bed, he puts himself at much higher risk for post-surgical complications like pneumonia and blood clots.

Your loved one will not be allowed to sit in the tub and bathe after the surgery, but he may take a shower. If it is hard for your loved one to get into the shower, sponge baths are also an option. Many pharmacies also sell dry shampoo that does not need to be rinsed out so individuals can keep their hair clean even if they cannot shower. Once the surgical staples are removed, wait for the doctor to give the green light for bathing to resume.

If your loved one still drives, he should be able to start driving his car about six weeks out from surgery. Again, wait for the doctor to give you the go-ahead before suggesting it. When your loved one is ready to start driving again, go online to your state's department of motor vehicles and print the form that will allow you to use handicapped parking spaces. Complete this form, get your doctor's signature and return it to the agency indicated on the form. Having the handicapped sticker will allow your loved one to park close to the entrance of a store or business so he doesn't have to walk far.

While non-impact activities like walking, swimming and stretching may be appropriate even immediately after surgery, discourage your loved one from doing high impact activities such as jogging or jumping rope. If you are in doubt about whether or not an activity is safe, check with your doctor or physical therapist.

Finally, pay careful attention to your loved one's pain level when he gets out of the hospital. Many older adults were raised to be stoic and not complain about discomfort, so you may need to ask, "Dad, on a scale from one to ten, with one being almost no pain, and ten being the worst pain you ever felt, where are you now?" Ask your doctor about the best ways to handle pain aside from medications.

Emotional Considerations. While having surgery is never fun, most people are hopeful going into knee replacement surgery. At the very least, they expect it to stop their pain; at best, they hope it will give them back a degree of mobility that they haven't had in years. Encourage your loved one to express his hopes to you. When and if he hits an emotional low after the surgery, gently remind him of all the reasons that the physicians, his family and he decided that surgery was such a good idea in the first place and what, optimally, the surgery will allow him to do with his life after recovery.

Abdominal Surgery

If a person has an obstructed bowel, an infected appendix, an abdominal tumor or gallstones, he or she may require surgery. Abdominal surgery is usually done by laparoscope rather than by the wide, easily infected incisions that were more common in years prior. Still, even laparoscopic surgery can be very draining of one's energy. This is especially true if, in addition to the surgery, he also requires difficult follow-up treatment like radiation or chemotherapy.

Home Care Considerations. In his 2005 article, "Improving the Outcomes of Major Abdominal Surgery in Elderly Patients," Albert Lowenfels, MD, reported that older patients tend to recuperate slowly after abdominal surgery. He found that most patients reported it was six to twelve weeks before they could complete even simple tasks like dress themselves, or even stand and walk independently. The patients who did regain their previous level of functioning after surgery generally took three to six months to do so. Even after six months, Dr. Lowenfels found that hand grip remained diminished, which indicated to him that the patient continued to suffer at least mild weakness.

If an older adult has had abdominal surgery, he or she will probably require a high degree of hands on physical care, from help getting in and out of the shower or bath to help preparing meals and completing basic household chores. To aid in the recuperation process, it may be a good idea to hire a caregiver from a private duty home care agency to assist him with activities of daily living, light housekeeping and cooking while he gets his strength back.

Emotional Considerations. Research indicates that there are two primary factors that influence how well an individual will heal after abdominal surgery: preoperative status and whether or not they suffer post-surgical complications. When the patients themselves were asked what made the biggest difference in their recoveries, the vast majority placed receiving social support and support from family members at the top of the list.

Make time to pay significant attention to your loved one as he recovers from his surgery. Remind him that healing takes time and that there are things he can do to help produce a good outcome, like following the doctor's orders about diet and exercise. Be there to offer support and let your loved one express his fears and concerns, demonstrating active listening skills. Try to arrange for your loved one's friends to visit him at home. If an individual attends a church, synagogue, or mosque, he or she might also welcome a visit from his clergy. Feeling surrounded by a whole community of loving, caring people may keep the recovering patient from becoming discouraged during the slow healing process after surgery.

The next several chapters will look at various diseases that commonly lead to hospitalizations and how you can best provide care for an individual with the diseases discussed once they return home from the hospital.

CHAPTER THIRTEEN
Heart Related Diseases

Heart disease is the number one cause of death in the United States and Canada. There are different types of heart disease. The most common is a narrowing or blocking of the coronary arteries, which carry blood to the heart. If the artery becomes completely blocked blood flow to the heart stops and heart muscle starts to die. This is what we have come to know as a heart attack, requiring immediate hospitalization and treatment.

Another type of heart disease occurs when the heart valves do not function correctly. Some people are born with valve damage; others develop it later in life. The valve problem about which you most commonly hear is mitral valve prolapse. In mitral valve prolapse, the valve doesn't close firmly after the heart pumps. This allows blood to leak back into the heart. If the condition is serious enough, it may lead to heart failure.

Heart failure is a third type of heart-related disease. Heart failure means that the heart simply doesn't pump well. Heart failure can lead to symptoms of fatigue, retaining fluid and experiencing a crippling shortness of breath. Heart failure can often be treated and controlled, but the only way to cure it is with a heart transplant.

Statistics/Demographics

According to the National Institute of Health, heart attacks and other forms of heart disease are most prevalent in men over 45 and women over 55. Other risk factors include smoking, high blood pressure, obesity, inactivity and diabetes.

Reasons for Hospitalization

The most common reason for a person to go into the hospital for heart disease is because he or she has suffered a heart attack, an interruption of blood to the heart muscle.

People with heart failure often come to the hospital after a "flare up" of their condition which leads them short of breath, extremely fatigued and often extremely frightened. Still others with heart disease may enter the hospital for a planned surgery such as a repair of the mitral valve or a heart transplant.

Home Care Physical Needs

If your loved one had a heart attack, doctors will probably recommend that she enroll in an inpatient or outpatient cardiac rehabilitation program. Cardiac rehab involves exercise training, education about the heart and keeping it healthy, stress reduction techniques and advice about controlling risk factors.

If your loved one had a flare up of congestive heart failure (CHF), she may come home close to her baseline, or her condition may have declined significantly. Before you leave the hospital, talk with the nurse and physical therapist about the kind of assistance your loved one will need at home. After a flare-up, the doctor may prescribe oxygen to help your loved one breathe easier.

If your loved one has been getting worse steadily, and the hospitalizations are coming closer and closer together, it might be a good idea to ask your doctor for a hospice referral. Hospice can keep your loved one comfortably at home and prevent future hospitalizations.

When she comes home from the hospital, you may need to provide light assistance with activities of daily living while any surgical wounds heal. As always, encourage your loved one to do as much as possible for herself. Any exercise—even the movement of getting dressed in the morning—is good.

Depending on the doctor's advice, encourage your loved one to get moderate exercise during the day. Suggest a walk around the home, or block if the individual is up to it. If the doctor approves, consider buying her a low cost treadmill so she can exercise easily.

The recovering patient will probably have to adhere to a strict cardiac diet which means decreased sodium, or salt, reduced calories and portions to reach and maintain a healthy weight, fewer fats, and a limit placed on other fluids, especially alcohol. While a home-delivered meals program is often a good choice for the older adult recuperating at home after a hospital stay, in the case of heart disease, it may not be helpful. Most home-delivered meals programs do not have the time to create special diets and many of the foods they serve may be on the patient's "forbidden" list.

Home Care Emotional Needs

Depending on the prognosis, the patient's reactions may vary from joy at having survived a heart attack to deep depression that a chronic illness is getting worse.

If she is thrilled just to be alive, share her relief and joy—you're probably thrilled to have her alive as well. Some people who have survived a heart attack may jump at the chance to educate themselves with information that will prevent them from having another one. Others may feel invincible ("See, the worst happened and it didn't kill me!") and desire to immediately return to their former lifestyle. If this is the case with your loved one, gently emphasize that she dodged a bullet and that the next heart attack is likely to be more debilitating unless she learns to follow the doctor's orders and take better care of herself. Perhaps the two of you could agree to eat healthier foods and exercise together.

Some people are terrified at the idea that they had a heart attack and are afraid to do anything that might provoke another. These people may sit around all day, not doing anything, terrified that the next attack is just around the corner. This kind of immobility coupled with anxious waiting can lead to depression. The best remedy for this emotional reaction is to arrange for your loved one to talk directly with the doctor about the things she can do to reduce her risk of another heart attack. If she is still terrified to move around, suggest small, easy projects such as helping you fold laundry or taking a walk across the street to visit a neighbor. Chances are that once your loved one is up, moving and enjoying life her fears will start to dissipate.

Some people who suffer a heart attack go into full cardiac arrest; this is when the heart has stopped and the brain stops receiving blood. Many people remember nothing about this time other than waking up in the hospital, but some people have what the literature refers to as NDEs or Near Death Experiences. These often involve seeing a beautiful bright light, reuniting with deceased family members or friends, reviewing their lives and finally being told that it isn't their time to go yet. No one is sure whether Near Death Experiences are spiritual or biological in nature, but if you know someone that has had an NDE and wants to talk about it, listen nonjudgmentally. Whatever its origin, the experienced episode can be life-changing.

If your loved one comes home after a worsening of congestive heart failure, she may simply seem tired and a little depressed. Encourage her to move around physically as much as the doctor allows, and remind her that even though she is suffering from a serious illness, she is still alive today and that is what matters. If your loved one expresses to you that she is tired of all the hospitalizations and is ready to die, talk to her doctor about involving hospice care.

Many family members find that their work and family commitments may not allow them to devote as much time as required with their loved one. In these situations, which are quite common, the individual benefits from having someone from a private duty home care agency come in a few hours a week to read to her, talk to her, help her with errands and do light housekeeping and cooking.

CHAPTER FOURTEEN
Cancer

Cancer occurs when abnormal or malignant cells begin to grow out of control in the body. Cancer can occur on almost any part of the body—in the brain, on the skin, in a major organ—some cancers respond well to treatments; others do not.

Some of the most common types of cancer include breast cancer, which occurs primarily in women, colon and rectal cancer, non-small cell lung cancer and prostate cancer.

Statistics/Demographics

According to the American Cancer Society, 1.6 million people in the United States are diagnosed with cancer every year. The Canadian Cancer Society cites an additional 180,000 Canadians are diagnosed with cancer each year. Seventy-five percent of cancers occur in people over the age of 55.

Prognosis

A person who has been diagnosed with cancer is often anxious about his prognosis, or how long he can live with the disease. The prognosis depends on many variables: where the tumor is located in the body, whether or not the malignancy is especially aggressive and the stage of the tumor. Very simply, the stage depends on the size of the tumor and how far it has spread. Stage I, for instance, usually means a small tumor that has not spread to adjacent lymph nodes or organs. Stage IV, on the other hand, indicates a tumor that has spread or metastasized to distant parts of the body.

Reasons for Hospitalization

Hospitalizations may occur at several points during cancer diagnosis and treatment. A person may be admitted into the hospital at the time he is diagnosed with cancer, especially if the cancer is causing disturbing symptoms and treatment needs to begin immediately. People receiving especially toxic types of chemotherapy may be routinely hospitalized so that the medicine can be given on an inpatient basis. People with cancer may also present to the hospital with complications resulting from the cancer spreading. Finally, patients who are close to death may be admitted to the hospital to die or to allow the discharge planner and her team to get plans for hospice in place.

Home Care Physical Needs

The home care cancer patient may be extremely active and mobile, or he may be exhausted by the treatments he is undergoing and/or the disease process. Talk with your doctor and with the nurse on the oncology unit to find out if there are any restrictions on your loved one's activities.

While it is a good idea to encourage self-sufficiency among those being treated for cancer, as long as the doctor approves, remember that extreme fatigue is a natural reaction to many types of cancer treatments. Individuals recovering from treatments may need to spend a lot of time sleeping and resting, especially in the days immediately following a treatment.

If your loved one will be returning from the hospital with new medical equipment such as a wheelchair, walker, cane or prosthetic device, check each room carefully for hazards resulting in a fall or accident like electrical cords that extend across the middle of the floor or throw rugs. Also check to be sure that the doors in the recently discharged patient's home are large enough to accommodate his wheelchair and his walker. Alert the discharge planner immediately if you find a problem.

If the individual's cancer is advanced, he or she may experience significant pain. Many older adults believe that expressing pain is a sign of weakness. Others are afraid that brining up pain with their medical team will distract the team from the "more important" medical concerns the individual has. If your loved one is unlikely to complain about his symptoms, watch him for non-verbal pain signals such as wincing, furrowing his brow, limping, or putting a hand up to cover the area that is painful. Ask your loved one to tell you about pain, adding that being in pain doesn't make him "weak" and that pain can be controlled to improve his quality of life.

Nutrition is another important area of focus for individuals with cancer. As long as your loved one is fighting cancer, he needs nutritious food to help him in the battle. If your loved one doesn't feel like eating, try getting him to drink nutritional supplements like Boost or Ensure. Some people who refuse to drink a nutritional supplement may be coaxed to take a few bites if the shake is mixed with ice cream.

If your loved one's illness does not respond to treatment, you may be faced with end of life care. If your loved one cannot or chooses not to receive any more curative treatment for his cancer, and if the doctor estimates that his life expectancy is six months or less, ask for a referral to a hospice program.

Hospice uses a multidisciplinary team comprised of a registered nurse/case manager, a licensed practical nurse, a hospice aide, a social worker, a chaplain and sometimes a volunteer to help you care for your loved one in his home. Hospice teams also are available to visit patients in an assisted living facility or a nursing facility. The hospice team can teach you the how to cope with an approaching death and how to keep your loved one physically, emotionally and spiritually comfortable during the last days of his life.

Home Care Emotional Needs

Not everyone reacts the same way to a cancer diagnosis. Some people come out fighting. Others give up and become profoundly depressed as soon as they hear the word cancer. Still others hold onto a certain amount of denial and refuse to talk about their diagnosis, even as they go through treatment.

If your loved one is struggling with depression after his diagnosis, encourage him to schedule a conference with his doctor. Ask your loved one's permission to attend the meeting as a second set of ears. If your loved one doesn't bring up his depression, bring up your concerns. The doctor may recommend counseling with a mental health professional, antidepressants, or both. More importantly, your doctor may be able to give your loved one information about his cancer that can ease his anxiety and depression.

If your loved one has been in the hospital for surgery or chemotherapy, you may be surprised to find that his mood when he gets home is quite upbeat, even if the treatments have altered his appearance or made him violently sick. Most people receiving treatment feel mentally positive because they feel that they are actively doing something positive to fight the cancer. Don, a man in his sixties with a luxurious head of hair didn't complain a bit when chemotherapy caused him to go bald. Asked why he didn't mind, he responded with a grin, "If that's what chemotherapy is doing to my hair follicles, just imagine the beating it's giving those cancer cells."

Ironically, people are more positive through the treatment than they are after treatment is completed. When they were being treated—even if the treatments made them sick—their mind was occupied with a sense that they were being proactive, taking charge of the cancer and giving it a beating as Don said. Patients who complete the treatment, or who are advised to "watch and wait" before they undergo any treatments contrastingly may feel a sense of anxiety and depression over a perceived belief that they are not doing anything to fight the disease. In reality, watchful waiting is a common and often beneficial approach that many patients are strongly advised to take in varying stages of the disease.

Another reason why individuals tend to get depressed after treatment is over is because many of the people they have counted on for support slip back into their old routines and the patient is left alone to deal with complicated feelings and fears. It is important to remember that individuals still require support, even after the treatment ends. Depending on what a cancer survivor can do physically, try to engage him in an activity he enjoyed before he was diagnosed with cancer, like bird watching or researching his family tree. If your loved one wants to talk about his feelings, listen empathetically and don't judge what he says–statements such as "what do you mean you're depressed? You should feel grateful!" can be hurtful to a cancer survivor.

If the news is bad and the treatment isn't helping, give your loved one all the emotional support you can. You don't have to talk about his feelings if that makes him uncomfortable. Sometimes sitting beside him and holding his hand is all you need to do. You can also help your loved one by encouraging him to review significant or humorous moments in his life. As your loved one grows more ill, don't be surprised if he pulls away from you a little. He isn't angry and you haven't done anything wrong. Detaching oneself from the living is an ordinary part of the dying process.

If the treatment puts the cancer into remission, your loved one's feelings may be complex. He may be relieved that the treatment worked. At the same time, he may worry that the cancer will come back. He may even experience some survivor guilt that he survived when some of the other cancer patients he met during treatment did not. Again, empathetic listening is the best gift you can offer your loved one as he struggles to make sense of this new, post-cancer world.

CHAPTER FIFTEEN
Stroke

Strokes are also known as cerebrovascular accidents or CVAs. There are two kinds of strokes. The first, called an ischemic stroke, occurs when an artery that supplies the brain with blood becomes blocked or clogged, cutting off the blood supply to a part of the brain. Denied of nourishment, brain cells quickly begin to die. Ischemic strokes account for 90 percent of strokes. The second type of stroke, the hemorrhagic stroke, occurs when a blood vessel in the head bursts or begins to leak blood, damaging the sensitive tissue of the brain.

Symptoms of stroke include sudden trouble walking or carrying out other routine tasks, slurred speech or difficulty understanding what others are saying, paralysis, tingling, or numbness on one side of the body or face, vision problems such as blurred vision or seeing double, and sudden, severe headaches.

Statistics/Demographics

Strokes are the third leading cause of death in the United States and account for approximately 7% of annual deaths in Canada. Around half a million people are diagnosed with strokes every year. Of those, 150,000 die immediately. The rest are left with varying degrees of impairment. There are millions of adults living with stroke-related brain damage. Two-thirds of strokes occur in people aged 65 or older.

Prognosis

The prognosis depends on several factors, including the type of stroke, the part of the brain damaged by the stroke, how quickly the person received treatment and the person's prior level of functioning.

Strokes that damage the left side of the brain result in impairment on the right side of the body. They also may damage the speech or language center of the brain, making communication difficult.

Strokes that damage the right side of the brain result in impairment on the left side of the body. They are also more likely to affect spatial skills.

Reasons for Hospitalization

Hospitalization commonly occurs following the onset of stroke symptoms. The patient is typically treated and observed in the hospital for a few days and is then referred to the most aggressive rehabilitation program she can tolerate.

Home Care Physical Needs

The individual's physical needs will depend on which part of the brain was damaged, how much damage occurred before treatment could be initiated and her ability to tolerate and benefit from a rehabilitation program.

Strokes may result in temporary or permanent paralysis to one side of the face or body, problems forming speech, understanding speech, or being able to express ideas, impulsivity and memory loss.

Encourage your loved one to do as much as possible for herself. Use verbal cues ("Put your left shoe on") and tactile cues (lightly touching the left foot) instead of stepping in to take over your loved one's care entirely. This requires extra time and patience, as it means waiting for your loved one to complete tasks that you know you could accomplish much faster. If you find yourself becoming frustrated, try to involve other family members in the care plan or hire a caregiver from a private duty home care agency.

Immediately following the stroke, your loved one will probably need someone to supervise and assist her with more complex tasks, such as money management, running errands, or preparing and eating a meal. Many communities or senior centers offer a nutritionally balanced home-delivered meal five days per week. For more information on home delivered meals and other services that are available to help older adults recuperate, contact your local Area Agency on Aging.

Home Care Emotional Needs

Studies suggest that anywhere from 30 to 60 percent of stroke victims become depressed following their stroke. This is partly due to frustration with physical limitations; it may also be a result of damage to the part of the brain that regulates mood. Symptoms of depression include sadness, tearfulness, withdrawing from activities previously enjoyed, lack of motivation, over eating or turning away food and sleeping too much or being unable to sleep. If you notice these symptoms, or if your loved one frequently makes statements about being "blue" or "down," talk to her doctor. Psychotherapy and medication are effective against most types of depression. You can also help by encouraging your loved one to work at her therapy program, praising her successes, and offering her as much independence and choice in her daily routine as possible.

If your loved one is able to leave the house, suggest that she attend a support group for stroke survivors. The hospital social worker can refer you to a local support group in the community.

Finally, some people undergo a noticeable change in personality, especially if the stroke damaged the frontal lobe of the brain which regulates impulse control. One woman, for instance, reported that after her normally shy and reserved mother suffered a stroke, she started "using cusswords" and even angrily ordered a doctor out of her room.

It's fine to provide reminders about appropriate behavior ("Mom, some people get offended when they hear that language in public") as long as you don't shame or scold your loved one. Remember that her behavior is not currently under her control and try not to be embarrassed and to maintain a positive attitude in the event that a public outburst does occur.

CHAPTER SIXTEEN
Diabetes

Diabetes is a condition which affects the way our bodies produce and use insulin. Normally when we eat, the cells in our body use the sugars in the food for energy. Insulin is a substance manufactured by the pancreas that acts like a key to "unlock" the cells so that they can utilize the sugars. If our bodies don't produce insulin, or if the insulin we produce is no longer able to unlock the cells, the cells become starved for energy. At the same time, the sugar that the cells can no longer access builds up in the body and causes damage to the tissues and organs.

There are two types of diabetes. Type I occurs when the pancreas simply stops making insulin. This type of diabetes is usually diagnosed in childhood. Type II diabetes occurs when the insulin produced by our bodies is no longer able to unlock the cells. Type II diabetes is often preceded by a condition called insulin resistance.

Statistics/Demographics

There are 27 million individuals living with diabetes in the United States and Canada. Each year, approximately 2 million new cases are diagnosed in adults over the age of 20. Diabetes affects more men than women.

Prognosis

In 2010, diabetes was listed as an underlying or contributory cause of death on over 200,000 death certificates. People with poor blood glucose control are more likely to suffer heart disease, strokes, high blood pressure, vision loss, kidney disease, damage to the nervous system and lower limb infections and amputations.

Reasons for Hospitalization

There are several reasons why a person with diabetes might require hospitalization. By the time diabetes is diagnosed, its victims are often suffering from hyperglycemia or dangerously high blood sugar levels. Symptoms of hyperglycemia include headache, a constant sensation of feeling thirsty and irritability. People with hyperglycemia may need to be hospitalized for care and observation while their blood sugar levels are brought under control. People with a new diagnosis of diabetes usually meet with a diabetes wellness educator to discuss medications and lifestyle changes they can make to achieve blood glucose control.

People who inject insulin to treat their diabetes are also vulnerable to hypoglycemia, or blood glucose levels that are too low. Symptoms of hypoglycemia include dizziness, trembling, sweating and confusion. Hypoglycemia can usually be treated outside of the hospital by eating or drinking something to elevate the blood sugar levels such as hard candy, a few tablespoons of peanut butter, a small packet of sugar dissolved in warm water, or a glass of chocolate milk. If hypoglycemia is not treated promptly, the person may lapse into a coma and die.

Diabetics may also require hospitalization for infections such as pneumonia or influenza. Another reason for hospitalization is an infected wound on the feet or lower legs. Because people with diabetes often suffer from impaired circulation, wounds to the lower extremities do not heal well and may become infected, a condition called cellulitis. Due to nerve damage, a person with diabetes may not feel pain to alert him that something is wrong.

If cellulitis is allowed to continue without treatment, it may lead to sepsis, or an infection that is carried by the bloodstream throughout the body. Some diabetics require amputation of their toes, feet, or lower legs to treat wounds that have become gangrenous.

Home Care Physical Needs

If your loved one has recently been diagnosed with diabetes, you and he may both need education about the medications he is to take, if any, and how and when to check his blood glucose levels.

Just a few years ago, people with diabetes were forbidden to eat any sweets. This forced diabetics with a sweet tooth to "sneak" their favorite foods, a practice which resulted in distrust between the patient and his health team and poor blood glucose control. Today, dietitians and diabetes educators work with patients to incorporate small portions of their favorite foods into their diet so that it is realistic and manageable. Still, it should be emphasized that carefully watching what one eats remains an important element in regulating blood glucose levels. The American Diabetes Association recommends a diet with plenty of fruits, green leafy vegetables, whole grains, lean meats and fish and low or nonfat dairy items.

If you're cooking for a diabetic, you also need to take portion size into consideration. Restaurants typically serve portions of food that are much larger than a single serving size and we get accustomed to eating more food than we actually need. Since eating too much of even the right foods can lead to weight gain, it's important to get an idea of what a single serving of food looks like. For instance, a single serving of meat is no larger than a deck of cards, and a serving of milk is eight ounces, or about one-fourth the size of a large soda. When in doubt, go by the rule that a serving of food is usually no larger than a clenched fist.

In addition to watching his diet, your loved one will also benefit from regular exercise. Even walking around the block or spending some time on a stationary bicycle while watching television will help.

Another aspect of a diabetic's physical care is foot care. Because of the heightened risk of infection of the legs and feet, any foot problems, even something as simple as an ingrown toenail, should be treated by a podiatrist, a doctor who specializes in foot care.

Check his feet and legs at least once a week for injuries such as cuts, scratches and abrasions and notify his doctor if anything seems out of the ordinary. Don't assume you will hear a complaint if he is injured. Diabetics frequently suffer from a condition called neuropathy, or damage to the nerves, that diminish sensations in the feet and legs. Your loved one could have a badly infected cut and not even be aware of it.

If a diabetic does have an injury that becomes infected, the doctor may arrange for him to receive home health services so that a nurse can help treat the wound and make sure that it heals properly.

You can help prevent injuries by making sure that your loved one's shoes fit properly and by discouraging going barefoot. A heavy pair of slippers or socks with non-slip soles is an excellent investment.

Home Care Emotional Needs

It is not uncommon for people to become anxious or depressed after being diagnosed with diabetes. This is especially true if the doctor is asking them to make significant lifestyle changes quickly. Doctors who received training several years ago may not be aware of the more lenient dietary guidelines for diabetics, so encourage your loved one to ask for a referral to a diabetes wellness educator or a registered dietitian who is trained in working with diabetics.

Another helpful intervention for the depression and anxiety that sometimes accompanies a diabetic diagnosis is attending a support group. The hospital social worker can refer patients to a diabetes support group that meets locally. Your loved one may find it reassuring and informative to talk with other diabetics who have adjusted well to living with the illness.

Finally, it's important to realize that your loved one's mood may be a clue as to his physical condition. If he is unusually irritable or easily angered, for instance, his blood glucose levels may be too high, and if he seems anxious or shaky, his blood glucose levels may be too low. Encourage your loved one to become aware of the link between blood glucose levels and mood so that he does not feel out of control or at the mercy of feelings he does not understand.

CHAPTER SEVENTEEN
Alzheimer's Disease and Related Dementias

Dementia is the term used to describe a constellation of cognitive symptoms such as short- and long-term memory loss, impaired decision-making ability, inability to recognize everyday objects, poor impulse control and difficulty planning and completing a task like going to the bathroom or getting dressed.

The most common cause of dementia is Alzheimer's disease, a condition which causes plaques and tangles in the nerve cells of the brain. Other common causes of dementia include vascular dementia (a dementia caused by reoccurring small strokes), late stage Parkinson's, long-term alcohol abuse, dementia with Lewy Bodies and front temporal dementia.

Statistics/Demographics

Age is the greatest risk factor for developing dementia, although early-onset Alzheimer's has a strong genetic link. According to the Alzheimer's Association, nearly 5.4 million people in the United States and 500,000 people in Canada are living with a diagnosis of Alzheimer's or a related dementia. Additionally, one in eight people over the age of 65 and one half of people over the age of 85 experience dementia symptoms. Two-thirds of the people currently living with Alzheimer's disease are women.

Because the population in North America is aging at the fastest rate in history, the number of people living with Alzheimer's disease is predicted to double by the year 2050.

Prognosis

Alzheimer's is considered a terminal disease, though it may progress very slowly. People who have been diagnosed with Alzheimer's disease may survive as few as two years or as many as twenty years.

Alzheimer's can kill by damaging the brain until people no longer remember how to perform basic life functions such as swallowing and breathing. In many cases, though, death comes when older people experience complications of dementia such as aspiration pneumonia (a lung infection that occurs when food is inhaled into the lungs) or a serious fall.

Reasons for Hospitalization

Alzheimer's disease in itself does not necessitate hospitalization, but people with dementia may be hospitalized after developing infections like pneumonia, influenza or even urinary tract infections. Dementia also makes people more vulnerable to falls and hospitalization may occur after a fall that results in a broken bone or head injury.

A patient with Alzheimer's may also be hospitalized after wandering away from home and suffering frostbite, heatstroke, dehydration or injury.

Finally, some Alzheimer's patients come to hospital emergency rooms with injuries that cannot be easily explained. Because people with dementia can be exhausting to care for and are therefore at a higher risk for being abused or neglected, a person with a suspicious injury may be hospitalized until the medical staff is positive that the patient is being discharged into a safe environment.

Home Care Physical Needs

The amount of physical care an Alzheimer's patient requires depends on the stage of the illness. A person experiencing early to mid-stage Alzheimer's symptoms may show significant cognitive impairment but very little physical impairment. This can make caring for your loved one challenging. As the exasperated wife of one Alzheimer's patient said after her husband wandered away from home, "It's like trying to take care of a two-year old who is bigger than I am."

The greatest physical risks to patients in the earlier stages of dementia include falling, wandering and injuring oneself at home.

It's practically impossible to guarantee that you will prevent your loved one from falling. Even skilled nursing facilities that offer dementia care units cannot promise that their patients will never fall. You can reduce the likelihood of falls by removing throw rugs, making sure the patient's shoes have non-slip soles, installing grab bars and non-slip mats in the bathroom and bathtub and by making sure that your loved one uses a walker or cane if the doctor has recommended that she do so.

People experienced in Alzheimer's care often say that it's not a question of if an Alzheimer's patient will wander—it's a question of when. Wandering, also referred to as elopement, may occur for many different reasons. People with dementia become confused about time and space. They may forget the layout of the house they've lived in for thirty years. Thus, a person trying to get to the bathroom in the middle of the night may become confused, wander out the front door and be unable to find her way back inside.

Being unable to recognize familiar surroundings is a scary experience for the Alzheimer's patient. Many people with Alzheimer's disease ask their caregivers to take them "home," even if they are at home. They may wander around the house, desperately looking for the door that will take them back to an environment that they remember and feel comfortable in. All too often, they find a door leading to the outside instead.

Your loved one may also wander if she gets confused while taking a walk in the neighborhood. Ruth, an Alzheimer's patient who had lived with her daughter for almost ten years, used to go out and pick up the paper every morning. Her daughter thought it was a good way for her to enjoy being outside and get a little exercise. She never dreamed this behavior could put Jenny in harm's way. One morning, Ruth went out to get the paper as usual and didn't return. Her daughter found her wandering several blocks away, still holding the paper in one hand. Ruth had forgotten which house belonged to her daughter.

Like falls, wandering cannot always be prevented, but there are steps you can take to reduce its likelihood and minimize the danger should it occur. One inexpensive measure you can take is to add a chain lock to each outside door. Install the lock away from the doorknob and below or above your loved one's eye level so that she is unlikely to notice it. Chances are she will not be able to figure out how to undo the lock.

You can also purchase a door alarm which beeps loudly when a door is opened. The noise will alert you when your loved one is trying to exit the house and it may startle her away from the door as well.

Another simple way to help keep your loved one safe is to disguise outside doors with wallpaper, or to place large red signs on them that say "STOP" or "DO NOT ENTER."

These ideas may seem overly simplistic, but a confused, disoriented person usually cannot figure out tricky locks and door alarms and will hesitate to disobey a sign that forbids entrance.

Just in case your loved one does make it out the door, you can take certain steps to reduce the likelihood that she will become lost or injured. If your neighbors do not already know your loved one, take her to their doors and introduce her to them. Explain to your neighbors that your loved one is forgetful and that if they see her outside without you, they should call you immediately. Then provide a phone number where you can be reached easily as well as the phone numbers of some other family members who can intervene if you can't be reached.

For a yearly fee, you can also enroll your loved one in the Alzheimer's Association's Safe Return program. The Safe Return program provides a durable bracelet for the individual to wear. Information on the bracelet includes a name or nickname, an identification number, a notice that your loved one suffers from a cognitive disorder and a toll-free phone number that a professional rescuer or a Good Samaritan can call if they find your loved one alone.

For a minimal fee, you can also get a bracelet that identifies you as a caregiver, so that if you should experience a medical emergency, the rescue personnel will know to look out for your loved one as well.

Another danger to be aware of is the risk of injury at home due to burns, scalding or ingesting toxic substances. Most burns occur in the kitchen during meal preparation. If your loved one likes to help you with meals, steer her towards tasks like setting the table or peeling potatoes that keep her away from the stove and oven. Cigarettes are another source of fire and burn injuries. Make sure that your loved one does not have access to cigarettes or to a lighter unless you or another caregiver is nearby to supervise her. Talk to her doctor about prescribing a nicotine patch to help her through withdrawal symptoms. Also, be aware that for many people with Alzheimer's, out of sight really is out of mind. If you confiscate the cigarettes without making a fuss about it, your loved one may forget about them entirely.

Scalding injuries can occur in the kitchen when a confused person accidentally tips a pan with hot fluids. Another source of scalding injuries is hot tap water. Lowering the temperature on your hot water thermostat can significantly reduce the risk of scalding injuries while washing hands, bathing, or showering.

Home Care Emotional Needs

Depression is often a problem for people with dementia. It may occur immediately after diagnosis or after an individual suspects he or she has a cognitive problem. An Alzheimer's diagnosis is devastating news, especially to someone who has always valued being "sharp," and in the earliest stages of Alzheimer's, your loved one may be acutely aware of her declining abilities. The Alzheimer's Association offers online support for people who are aware of their diagnosis; some local chapters also offer face-to-face support groups.

You can help by listening supportively as your loved one discusses her thoughts, feelings and concerns around this disease. You can also help your loved make arrangements with which she feels comfortable. This might include helping her find a financial planner to make sure her money is secure or an elder care lawyer to draw up legal documents such as a living will or durable powers of attorney for healthcare and financial purposes. Try to respect the person's wishes, even if the requests seem strange or even morbid.

One man, for instance, asked his brother to take him around to different nursing homes so he could decide in advance where he would go if he could no longer be cared for at home and a woman insisted that her husband take her to the local funeral parlor so she could discuss her final wishes with the funeral director. Both felt much better for having made these arrangements while they were still cognitively able.

During this time, it may be tempting to promise your loved one anything to calm her fears. ("Of course I won't put you in a nursing home, Mom.") While it is likely your loved one will not remember these promises at a later time, family members who have made them may feel guilty or ashamed if they have to go back on their word down the road. Instead of making a promise you may not be able to keep, it's better to say something like, "No one knows the future, Mom, but I promise I will take care of you here at home as long as I can."

Depression may also become a problem later in the disease process, long after your loved one has lost all self-awareness to recognize her decline. Depression that occurs later in the disease process is usually caused by chemical changes in the brain. This type of depression usually responds well to antidepressant medications. It also helps if you can maintain a calm, soothing attitude.

Anxiety is also an issue for many people with dementia. Some people are afraid without knowing why. Others may worry about needing to get "home," even if they are home. Still others will focus on fulfilling a past responsibility, thinking they have to go to work or pick the children up from school. Dementia patients who are anxious often ask the same question or make the same comment over and over.

This behavior can stretch a caregiver's patience to the breaking point. It may help to remember that your loved one isn't doing this on purpose. She does not remember that she asked, and you answered, the same question only a few seconds ago. Her brain is "stuck" in a groove much like a scratched vinyl record. To get her unstuck, try focusing her attention on another topic like listening to music, watching a television program she enjoys or looking at family pictures.

There may be times when the best response involves "therapeutic deception," or going along with your loved one's reality. If your loved one asks why her mother hasn't come for her, for instance, avoid saying, "Your mother has been dead for twenty years." A blunt response like this can create fresh grief and anxiety. It's better to engage in what is called "therapeutic lying" and provide a response that will calm your loved one, "I'm imagine she'll be along soon," or "I think she's running late today. Why don't you help me bake this pie until she gets here?"

Lisa, who took care of her aunt with Alzheimer's disease, remembers how shocked she was when her aunt did not remember the death of her husband, Lisa's uncle. "The first time she asked me where George was, I blurted out that George had died three years ago. Aunt Laurie cried for the rest of the day. The next time she asked, I said, 'Oh, I imagine he's still at work.' She nodded and that was the end of it."

Another emotional issue for people with dementia is paranoia. It's not unusual for people with dementia to accuse their caregivers of stealing from them or even hurting them physically. Statements like this can be very hurtful when you're trying your best to help your loved one.

Perhaps even harder to deal with is your loved one making such accusations against another caregiver. On the one hand, you want to protect your loved one if abuse or neglect is occurring; on the other hand, you're aware that her version of reality is not always objective reality. If you trust the other caregiver, talk with him or her about the accusations and try to figure out from where they may be originating.

CHAPTER EIGHTEEN
Parkinson's Disease

Parkinson's is a neurological disorder, a disease that attacks the nervous system which affect how a person moves. Symptoms of Parkinson's disease include tremors, walking with a shuffling gait or "freezing" while walking, inability to show facial expression, rigid muscles, loss of automatic movements such as swinging your arms when you walk, speech that is soft or slurred and, in some cases, dementia.

These symptoms are primarily caused by low levels of two neurotransmitters, dopamine and norepinephrine. Neurotransmitters are substances that enable the nerve cells of the brain to communicate with each other. Another change in the brains of some people with Parkinson's disease is the appearance unusual "clumps" of protein called Lewy Bodies. The presence of Lewy Bodies has been linked to dementia symptoms.

Statistics/Demographics

According to the Parkinson's Disease Foundation and Parkinson Society Canada, over one million individuals in the United States and 100,000 individuals in Canada are currently living with Parkinson's. Approximately 70,000 new cases are diagnosed each year in these two countries. Age appears to be the greatest risk factor for developing Parkinson's disease—of those living with the disorder; only about four percent were diagnosed before the age of 50. Men are at 1.5 times greater risk of developing Parkinson's than women.

Prognosis

Parkinson's disease advances at different rates for different people. There is no way to tell how quickly symptoms may progress. Some people experience significant physical disability within a few years after diagnosis; others remain independent for years. The popular actor Michael J. Fox, for instance, has lived for more than a decade with Parkinson's and to date is still able to work as a performer.

Parkinson's disease is not considered fatal and does not affect life expectancy. In a few cases, secondary complications of advanced Parkinson's such as choking or inhaling food into the lungs (aspiration pneumonia) may cause premature death.

Reasons for Hospitalization

Parkinson's patients typically come to the hospital after suffering from a fall or after developing an infection like pneumonia or influenza.

Planned admissions for patients who have chosen to undergo surgery for deep brain stimulation are also not unusual.

Home Care Physical Needs

Many Parkinson's disease patients remain relatively independent long after diagnosis. Others have more trouble and require more physical assistance.

One of the most common and frustrating issues that people with Parkinson's experience is difficulty getting dressed and grooming themselves. Tasks like buttoning shirts, doing up zippers, handling a razor or a toothbrush, or even stepping into a pair of sweat pants require fine motor coordination that most Parkinson's patients lack. If your loved one has trouble with these activities of daily living, notify his doctor. The doctor may suggest that your loved one work with an occupational therapist to identify adaptive techniques and equipment.

Older adults with Parkinson's are also at risk for falls. People with Parkinson's often walk with a slow, shuffling gait. The shuffling increases the risk of tripping. Parkinson's patients may also "freeze" while they are walking. A physical therapist can provide you with useful tips for reducing the risk of falls in those with this disease. Common suggestions include standing up as straight as possible, making sure the heel hits the ground first with each step, being aware of one's center of gravity and using assistive devices (e.g., walker or cane) as prescribed. Gentle exercise programs like tai chi or yoga can reduce the risk of falls by improving strength, flexibility and awareness of the body.

An individual with Parkinson's may experience problems with constipation. This is partly a symptom of the disease, which slows the digestive tract. It may also be a side effect of some medications routinely used to treat Parkinson's disease. Encouraging your loved one to eat foods high in fiber can resolve this problem without the need for medical intervention. If your loved one is severely constipated and cannot find relief from home remedies, talk to his doctor and ask about the possibility of adding a laxative to his list of medications.

Rigid muscles are typical of Parkinson's disease, but they can also be a source of discomfort and annoyance. Gentle massage therapy can help relieve muscle tension and promote relaxation and a sense of wellbeing. Many patients with Parkinson's find that exercises in physical, occupational and speech therapy are extremely helpful in allowing them to regain functions they thought they had lost forever. It is important for individuals to consistently practice these exercises, however.

If you do not have the time to assist your loved one in his or her exercises, consider getting support from a nearby rehabilitation center or hiring a private duty caregiver.

Home Care Emotional Needs

Depression is a common reaction to a Parkinson's diagnosis. Nobody likes the idea of having a physically disabling condition. Many people find comfort in attending support groups; it allows them to see that they are not alone with their problems, encourages socializations and introduces them to helpful ideas for coping with day to day tasks.

One-on-one therapy is also helpful for people with Parkinson's disease, especially if the therapist is familiar with Parkinson's and can combine cognitive behavioral therapy, which has an excellent track record for alleviating depression, with life skills training to help your loved one adapt to his new reality.

In some cases, depression and anxiety occurs due to chemical changes in the brain. Medication works well to control these symptoms.

Some people with Parkinson's experience hallucinations, delusions or other psychotic symptoms. These symptoms are usually a side effect of medications that increase the supply of dopamine in the brain. If this occurs, let the doctor know what is going on as soon as possible, so he or she can adjust the medications.

Finally, maintaining a close, trusting relationship with his treatment team is essential for your loved one's physical and emotional wellbeing. If your loved one does not like someone closely involved in his care, he may be less likely to report significant symptoms or to ask for needed assistance. If a conflict between your loved one and his treatment team does arise, you can help by listening to both sides and attempting to mediate differences. In some cases, you may need to help your loved one transfer his care to another doctor.

CHAPTER NINETEEN
Arthritis

Arthritis is a loose term applied to any condition that causes inflammation of the joints. Joints are the parts of the body where bones meet. There are over 100 types of conditions that can be termed arthritis. Two of the most common types are osteoarthritis and rheumatoid arthritis.

Osteoarthritis occurs when the tissue that provides a cushion between two bones breaks down. This condition can leading to the painful sensation of bone rubbing against bone.

Rheumatoid arthritis is an autoimmune disease. For unknown reasons, the immune system, which is supposed to protect us from outside invaders such as bacteria, starts attacking cells in the body. The attacks are initially focused on the membranes that line the joints, although the disease may go on to attack the organs as well. A person with rheumatoid arthritis may experience pain throughout her body. The pain may be chronic, or it may recede for a while and then flare up again.

Statistics/Demographics

According to the Arthritis Foundation, over 4.6 million Americans, or one in five adults, were living with arthritis as of 2006. Arthritis is the leading cause of disability of people over the age of 15.

Prognosis

Although rheumatoid arthritis is not considered a fatal disease, the average life expectancy for individuals who have rheumatoid arthritis is slightly shorter than average. This reflects the reality that the autoimmune disease—and the treatments for it—may result in secondary complications such as infections that result in death.

Most types of arthritis do not shorten the life span, although they can disable sufferers and seriously impact quality of life.

Reasons for Hospitalization

According to the Arthritis Foundation, arthritis results in over 500,000 hospitalizations each year. A person may be admitted to the hospital following a flare-up of arthritis symptoms or a pain emergency. People with arthritis are also vulnerable to falling and injuries related to falling are another reason why someone with arthritis may be hospitalized.

Individuals with rheumatoid arthritis who take immune-suppressing drugs may need to be hospitalized to treat infections that their immune systems can no longer wipe out. Dehydration caused by diarrhea may be a result of some of the medications prescribed for different types of arthritis and may warrant hospitalization in a person whose health is already fragile. Finally, patients who choose to undergo hip or knee replacements will spend some time in the hospital after the procedure before returning home or going to rehabilitation.

Home Care Physical Needs

Some people with arthritis experience only mild symptoms and are able to manage their pain and complete their activities of daily living without assistance. Other people, though, experience significant pain and swelling in the joints and are unable to perform simple tasks such as dressing or bathing.

It is a point of pride for many people to remain independent as long as possible. When you talk to your loved one about her arthritis, make it clear that you have no intention of "taking over" and are merely offering your help. Gently ask your loved one questions about her routine and whether or not arthritis has hampered it. ("Your knees look so sore and swollen, Mom. How do you get around the grocery store?")

If your loved one is agreeable, hire a private duty home caregiver to visit once or twice a week and help your loved one with the tasks that give her the most trouble.

One of your chief concerns in caring for a loved one with arthritis is adequately managing her pain. This may be accomplished with over the counter medications known as non-steroidal anti-inflammatories (NSAIDS). Examples of these medications include aspirin and ibuprofen. Since these medications can irritate your loved one's stomach, it's best to speak to a doctor before initiating them for long-term use.

Pharmacies also sell arthritis creams which can be applied directly to the skin over the painful joint.

There are other measures to try that don't require the use of medication. Experiment with your loved one to see whether a hot pad or an ice pack applied to the sore joints helps alleviate the pain.

It may sound counter-intuitive, but light exercise that doesn't stress or jar the joints such as walking, swimming, or using a stationary bicycle can actually be good for your loved one. Over time, it may lead to weight reduction which can reduce osteoarthritis symptoms of the knees and hips. It also strengthens the muscles that support the painful joints, and promotes balance and flexibility.

Some studies have also suggested that natural supplements may ease arthritis pain. Two supplements that you often hear about are chondroitin and glucosamine. So far the research as to their effectiveness has shown mixed results at best, but the bottom line is that even if they don't help, they don't usually harm, either. Omega-3 fatty oils have also been correlated with reduced inflammation and may benefit arthritis sufferers. Remember to have your loved one check with her doctor before starting to use supplements.

Your loved one can create a valuable pain management tool by keeping a pain log. This involves writing down when pain occurs, how intense the pain is on a scale of one to ten, what might have caused it or made it worse, what didn't help the pain and what, if anything, did help. Have your loved one keep the pain log for a week or two and then review it with her doctor. Together, your loved one and her doctor can pinpoint the circumstances that led to increased pain (kneeling in the garden, sitting too long in the same position) so that your loved one can avoid them in the future. Your loved one may also gain some valuable insights on the interventions that typically ease pain when it flares up.

Finally, if your loved one's current healthcare team is not able to adequately control her discomfort, urge your loved one to ask for a referral to a pain management clinic or to a doctor who specialized in treating chronic pain.

Home Care Emotional Needs

Depression, anxiety and chronic pain seem to go hand in hand. Because depression tends to focus attention inward on the body and its aches and pains, it can actually intensify the pain your loved one is feeling, which in turn makes the depression worse. Without intervention, it can become a vicious cycle.

Your loved one may need medication to alleviate her depression and anxiety. As an added benefit, one class of antidepressants, tricyclics, have been shown to alleviate pain in some people. Learning relaxation techniques may also help ease painful symptoms that have been made worse by anxiety and depression.

Your loved one may also want to consider attending a support group for people with arthritis or chronic pain, or seeking help from a mental health counselor who specializes in chronic pain issues. The hospital social worker can provide you with resources.

Pain can make people feel helpless and out of control. Your loved one may feel that she has been betrayed by her own body. The Arthritis Foundation encourages people living with arthritis to view pain as an ally, a powerful signal that their body needs them to take some sort of positive action.

CHAPTER TWENTY
Lung-Related Disorders

Our lungs allow us to breathe in air. They then isolate the oxygen and release it into the bloodstream to nourish the cells in the body. Without the proper amount of oxygen, cells start to die quickly. There are some acute diseases, such as pneumonia and influenza that affect how well the lungs function. There are also many chronic diseases which can make breathing difficult. The most common include chronic obstructive pulmonary disease (COPD), asthma and tuberculosis. COPD is an umbrella term that refers to a chronic blockage of airflow in the lungs. Doctors now prefer to use COPD instead of the older diagnoses bronchitis and emphysema. Because COPD is the most common lung problem among older adults, the rest of the chapter will focus on it.

Statistics/Demographics

According to the American Lung Association, 13.1 million adults in the United States alone were living with COPD in 2008. Another 11 million adults showed clinical evidence of impaired lung function and probably qualified for a COPD diagnosis. The Public Health Agency of Canada reports that over 3 million Canadians cope with a serious respiratory disease like COPD. Between one-half and one-third of people with COPD reported difficulty performing daily functions such as working, keeping up the house, socializing with friends and family and even sleeping. The most common risk factor for COPD is smoking.

Prognosis

COPD is a leading cause of death in the United States and Canada. It claims the lives of slightly more women than men. Although COPD is irreversible and gets worse over time, healthcare professionals cannot adequately predict how quickly the disease will progress in any given person. Studies have shown that abstaining from smoking can prolong life as well as reduce distressing symptoms that impair the quality of life.

Death from COPD usually results from respiratory failure infections of the lungs, and related health problems such as heart failure.

Reasons for Hospitalization

According to the American Lung Association, COPD accounted for 700,000 hospitalizations in 2006. The most common diagnoses that led to hospitalization were COPD exacerbation, which occurs when COPD symptoms suddenly get worse, infections such as influenza or pneumonia, and co-morbidities, problems like heart disease that seem to go hand in hand with COPD.

Home Care Physical Needs

How much physical care your loved one needs depends on how far the COPD has progressed and on many other physical conditions he has. He may feel weak or tired on some or most days. Resist the temptation to do everything for him and instead encourage him to do as much as possible for himself.

As long as his doctor approves, it's also helpful to involve your loved one in light exercise such as walking. Staying physically active and in peak health can slow the progression of COPD. If your loved one does engage in some form of exercise, expect him to need frequent rest breaks. He will have good days when he hardly needs to rest at all and bad days when he can barely walk a few steps without pausing to rest.

Ask your loved one's doctor to refer him to a therapy program so that a physical therapist and an occupational therapist can visit the home and make suggestions that will help your loved one maintain his independence. An occupational therapist, for instance, might recommend attractive clothing that is easy to put on and to take off. A physical therapist may recommend a special kind of wheeled walker with a seat your loved one can use if he or she becomes exhausted while walking.

Work with your loved one to figure out if there are any conditions or environmental factors such as dust, pollen, the odor of strong cleansers or warm, humid weather that make his COPD worse. Try to help him avoid these irritants.

People with COPD tend to use a lot of calories simply because they are putting forth such an effort to keep breathing. Muscle weakness/wasting and significant weight loss may occur as the disease gets worse. To counter this problem, make sure your loved one is eating a healthy diet. It may help to talk to a nutritionist or a dietitian about food suggestions and calorie intake. If your loved one is not on a cardiac diet, call your local senior center or Area Agency on Aging to ask about their home-delivered meals program. This will ensure that your loved one gets at least one-third of the nutrition he needs each day without having to put forth the effort of planning and preparing a meal.

There are also a couple of areas of which to be aware if your loved one is on oxygen. The first is the danger of tripping over the oxygen tubing. Since no one wants to feel restricted to just one room in his house, oxygen companies often deliver long lengths of tubing so your loved one can have some freedom of motion. The only problem with the long tubing is that it is easy to get one's feet tangled up in it and trip or fall. The good news is that most people who have been on oxygen for even a few days become experts at stepping over and around the tubing. For the first week or so, though, keep a vigilant eye on your loved one. If you notice the tubing getting tangled around his feet, tell him to stop walking and help him straighten it out.

Another risk related to oxygen is the risk of fire. This risk is magnified when you consider that many people continue to smoke even after being diagnosed with COPD. There's a common misconception that the oxygen will explode if it comes into contact with flames. It won't, but it can cause a fire that can burn your loved one's face and cause further damage to his already delicate respiratory system. In a worst case scenario, the fire can spread throughout the home and cause damage to your property.

If your loved one resists your attempts to make him quit smoking, the next approach is to tell your loved one that you want him to smoke safely. This means when he wants a cigarette, he needs to take his oxygen off, turn off the oxygen concentrator and go outside or into another room. This will prevent oxygen-fueled fires. As a fringe benefit, your loved one may be so disgusted with the whole procedure that he stops smoking voluntarily.

If your loved one has made giving up smoking a goal, talk to his doctor. The doctor may prescribe a nicotine patch or oral medication that can ease your loved one through the first few days of physical withdrawal.

Home Care Emotional Needs

The most common emotional reaction among people with lung problems is anxiety. Feeling like you can't catch your breath is terrifying. People who are especially anxious may hyperventilate, or take fast, shallow breaths that put even more stress on the lungs. You can help your loved one during these panicky moments by remaining calm and urging him to take slow, deep breaths. Breathing in through the nose and out through the mouth is especially helpful.

Sometimes people who are anxious can behave in manipulative ways. Their behavior makes sense in an odd sort of way—they have lost control of so much, it's natural for them to want to control their environment and the behavior of people around them, even if this means resorting to threats ("Go if you want to, but don't be surprised if you come back in the morning and find me dead."), passive aggressive behavior or trying to play two people against each other.

It can be easy to lose your temper with a loved one who is resorting to these tactics. Take a deep breath and remember he's trying to get his basic needs met the best he knows how.

Look at the real fears and concerns that underlie the tactics, and when you respond, speak directly to those concerns. For instance, rather than argue about whether or not your father will actually die if you leave him alone for a few hours, you might say something like, "Dad, I hear that you really don't want to be alone. I wish I could stay with you, but I have to work. Maybe we could hire someone to come in during the times when I have to be gone."

It's also a good idea to have a word with your loved one's doctor if your loved one seems anxious and fearful. Certain medications can alleviate anxiety and can provide both you and your loved one with a greater sense of peace of mind.

CHAPTER TWENTY-ONE
Kidney Disease

The kidneys help remove fluid and waste products from the body. They also help control the levels of certain substances in the body, release hormones that control blood pressure and produce Vitamin D. Some problems with the kidneys, like kidney stones, are time-limited, though painful, and are not life threatening.

Chronic kidney disease (CKD), also known as chronic renal failure (CRF), is a far more serious problem. Chronic kidney disease is an umbrella term used to cover a variety of conditions that damage the kidneys so they can no longer perform their most important functions.

Chronic kidney disease is often a result of diabetes or untreated high blood pressure. Early detection and treatment can help slow the progression of CKD. If chronic kidney disease becomes advanced before it is diagnosed, it may quickly develop into a condition called end stage renal disease, or ESRD, a life-threatening complication which requires dialysis or a kidney transplant.

Statistics/Demographics

According to the National Kidney Foundation, 26 million Americans are living with chronic kidney disease. The groups most at risk for developing this condition include African Americans, Pacific Islanders, Native Americans, and older adults of all races.

Prognosis

People with chronic kidney disease are more likely to have heart attacks and strokes than the general population.

Of the patients who go on dialysis, only 32% survive five years or more. Elderly patients and patients with diabetes typically have the worst outcomes.

The two year transplant survival rate, however, is 88 to 90 percent, making transplant a very desirable treatment among people with struggle with end stage kidney disease.

Reasons for Hospitalization

Diagnosing kidney problems can be tricky. By the time a diagnosis is confirmed, the patient may already be suffering the toxic effects of wastes building up in the body. Therefore, many patients are admitted to the hospital for emergency dialysis at the time of diagnosis. These patients may or may not need to continue on dialysis once the medical team has introduced diet changes and medications to protect the kidneys.

People may also require hospitalization if they become violently ill during a dialysis treatment.

Since patients with chronic kidney disease are at a higher risk for heart attacks and strokes, they may need to be hospitalized if these conditions occur.

Finally, some people with end stage kidney disease will skip one or more dialysis treatments and require emergency dialysis in the hospital. Missing treatments may indicate rebellion against the treatment, poor planning (for instance, not arranging for necessary transportation), or events beyond the person's control (for instance, a flood cutting off access to the clinic).

Home Care Physical Needs

Whether or not your loved one with chronic or end stage kidney disease depends on her age and on any secondary physical conditions she may experience. For instance, a kidney patient who has had a severe stroke may require almost total care, while someone who has remained relatively healthy may require no assistance with personal care at all.

The dietary needs of the patient with chronic kidney disease may be somewhat unusual and may even seem counter-intuitive. Instead of being told to drink eight glasses of water a day, for instance, your loved one's fluids will be restricted. Proteins are also to be avoided. If you have questions about what your loved one can and can't eat or drink, talk to her doctor and ask for a referral to a nutritionist or dietitian who specializes in the treatment of kidney disease.

Your loved one's doctor may also tell her to avoid certain over-the-counter drugs like laxatives which contain magnesium or aluminum, non-steroidal anti-inflammatory drugs (NSAIDs) and decongestants.

Aside from keeping an eye on your loved one's diet and medications, you may also need to help with practical matters such as arranging transportation if your loved one requires dialysis at a clinic or assisting your loved one with completing dialysis treatments at home. If the doctor suggests in-home dialysis, request a referral to a home health program so that a nurse can come to the house to provide teaching and monitoring until you and your loved one get the hang of how it works.

Home Care Emotional Needs

As with most chronic and potentially life-threatening diseases, it is not uncommon for a person to become depressed after the diagnosis of chronic kidney disease. Your loved one may benefit from antidepressants, psychotherapy, attending a support group, or going to a life skills program that will teach her how to manage her condition and remain as healthy as possible. The hospital social worker can help you access all of these resources. If she goes to a dialysis clinic, the social worker there can provide mental health screenings, supportive counseling and referrals to other mental health professionals as warranted.

After being on dialysis for a while, some people express the desire to stop the treatment. If your loved one expresses this wish, try to remain calm and encourage her to talk about why she wants the dialysis to stop. There are several possibilities.

There may be something your loved one dislikes about the dialysis center. Brendan, for instance, a dialysis patient in his forties with a mild developmental disability, announced to his mother that he would not go back to dialysis. His mother and the dialysis social worker spoke to him together and determined that Brendan often got bored during dialysis treatments. Furthermore, he thought the room was too cold. To remedy this situation, his family members bought him a laptop so he could watch his favorite movies during treatment and the social worker was able to find a warm blanket. Brendan never mentioned wanting to stop dialysis again.

Another reason why some people want to stop dialysis is that they are rebelling against the strict treatment plan that they must follow. The patients who rebel are often younger people who were in good health prior to their diagnosis. Often they are testing the waters, unable to believe that their body has completely betrayed them. If you think your loved one is in rebellion, a talk with the doctor is recommended. The doctor can explain that the medical consequence of stopping dialysis is death and usually occurs within a week or two after the last treatment. Since most people who are rebelling don't want to die, they will often agree to resume treatment. It may help if you and your loved one sit down together and make two lists: one of things she can't control and one of things that she can control. Encourage your loved one to exert control whenever possible. The choices can be as simple as what she wears, whether she wants to drive herself to the dialysis clinic or be driven and which of two foods in her recommended diet she would rather eat.

Another reason for refusing treatment is depression. As long as your loved one is alert, oriented and able to make decisions, she has the right to refuse a treatment, even if it would prolong or sustain her life. The problem with making a decision while profoundly depressed is that your loved one is only seeing part of the picture—the negative part. If you witness signs of depression such as tearfulness, withdrawing from people, losing interest in activities that were once enjoyed and disruptions with sleeping and eating, encourage your loved one to accept assistance from a mental health professional. Remind her that she may not be thinking clearly at the moment and that she can always decide to stop dialysis if she still wants to when the depression has lifted. Again, involve the doctor and the dialysis clinic social worker in these discussions.

Finally, the individual may have decided that his or her quality of life on dialysis is not acceptable. She may prefer death to continuing treatments that are often exhausting and may lose their effectiveness within a few years. You may hate your loved one's decision and disagree with it completely, but as long as she is cognitively intact, it is her decision to make. Having hospice involved during your loved one's final days may be helpful to both of you. Talk to the doctor and the hospice team so that you and your loved one will know what symptoms she might experience and how they can best be controlled. Hospice can usually sign your loved one up for services the day after the final dialysis treatment takes place.

CHAPTER TWENTY-TWO
Liver Disease

The liver plays a vital role in many life functions such as absorbing nutrients from food and clearing toxic substances from the body. Like kidney disease, liver disease is a generic term used to describe many conditions that damage the liver. These conditions may be genetic, or they may be caused by an illness such as hepatitis, or by the liver being over-exposed to alcohol, street drugs and certain prescription medications.

Common symptoms of liver problems include jaundice or yellowing of the whites of the eyes and the skin, abdominal pain and swelling due to the buildup of fluids (ascites), itching all over the body and unusual tiredness.

The most common, non-reversible diagnosis of liver disease is cirrhosis, or extreme scarring of the liver. People with cirrhosis are at risk of developing infections such as pneumonia or influenza. They may also experience malnutrition because the liver can no longer absorb nutrients and internal bleeding.

Statistics/Demographics

No one is sure exactly how many people are currently living with cirrhosis, but doctors estimate that 75 to 80 percent of cirrhosis cases could have been prevented by eliminating alcohol abuse. There are also 30 million adults living with hepatitis C, another condition that can cause scarring and damage to the liver.

Prognosis

In 2009, liver disease was the primary diagnosis in over 30,000 deaths in the United States and Canada. How long a person can survive with liver disease depends on several factors including the underlying cause of the cirrhosis, the health status before diagnosis and whether or not the patient adheres to his treatment plan.

Reasons for Hospitalization

In 2009, liver disease accounted for over 100,000 hospitalizations. Causes of hospitalizations in people with liver disease include complications of the disease such as ascites or internal bleeding and infections like pneumonia. Some people with liver disease who are in treatment for a drinking problem are admitted to the hospital for medical detoxification. A final reason for hospital admission is undergoing a liver transplant.

Home Care Physical Needs

Many people with liver disease are able to care for themselves without assistance. If the disease is very advanced and the individual is experiencing complications, however, he may need assistance with personal care. If you are unable to assist with caregiving duties, it may be a good idea to hire a private duty caregiver to assist with meal preparation to provide companionship, especially if the individual is starting eliminate or reduce alcohol consumption.

Dietary recommendations for people with liver disease include a diet low in sodium and high in fresh fruits and vegetables. Diet may be an especially important area of concern if the individual is struggling with an alcohol problem. People who are addicted to alcohol often suffer from poor nutrition. If in doubt about the best diet to provide for someone with liver disease, ask the person's doctor for a referral to a registered dietitian or nutritionist who is familiar with the treatment of liver disease.

One of the chief functions of the liver is clearing toxins from the body. When the liver begins to fail, these toxins can build up and cause changes in cognition and mood. Therefore, ask your doctor before giving your loved one any over-the-counter medication. If your loved one is being treated by several doctors, be sure to let them know about your loved one's liver disease diagnosis. It's also a good idea to mention it to the pharmacist who fills your loved one's prescriptions.

Home Care Emotional Needs

Be aware that if a person suddenly seems confused, disoriented and angry or irritable, this sudden change in status could be caused by toxins building up in the blood. This is a medical emergency—contact a physician or call 911 so he can receive the treatment he needs as fast as possible.

Doctors estimate that anywhere from 75 to 80 percent of the cirrhosis cases they see are related to alcohol abuse. If a person suffers from this problem, don't badger him, but offer him support and encouragement to abstain from alcohol or even to cut back on the amount he drinks. If he expresses interest in receiving substance abuse treatment, offer to help him find referrals. Talking to the hospital social worker is a great place to start.

Resource Corner: The Alcoholics Anonymous website (www.aa.org) serves the United States and Canada as an educational resource and source of information on local meetings.

Be aware that if your loved one drinks every day, he is likely to go through withdrawal symptoms such as seizures, nausea and vomiting if he stops cold turkey. Even otherwise healthy people have died as a result of severe withdrawal. Your loved one's health is already fragile, so if you think withdrawal will be an issue, help him admit himself to the hospital or find an inpatient substance abuse treatment center where he can be monitored and given medications to reduce unpleasant symptoms.

Mental health professionals estimate that anywhere from 15 to 30 percent of substance abuse addicts also have an underlying mental health problem such as depression. Depression is also common in people with chronic physical illnesses. If your loved one has a dual diagnosis (alcohol abuse plus an additional psychiatric disorder), he needs to receive treatment for both problems. Treatment for depression can include medication, depending on whether or not his doctor thinks he is healthy enough to tolerate it. Another treatment option is psychotherapy. Psychotherapy, especially in the form of Cognitive Behavioral Therapy (CBT), has proven to be effective in the treatment of depression. A support group for patients with liver disease is another possible source of help. If your loved one is still able to get up and around, encourage him to adopt an exercise program and remain as active as possible. Many studies show that exercise can treat depression as well as medications.

Finally, if your loved one's disease is alcohol-related, he may experience a lot of anger and self-blame. Listen supportively while he expresses his feelings. He may not need you to make any comment or offer any advice at all. If your loved one does ask you for reassurance, you can emphasize that you are proud of the efforts he or she is making to stay healthy now.

CHAPTER TWENTY-THREE
Psychiatric Disorders

Psychiatric disorders, sometimes referred to as mental disorders or mental illnesses, encompass well over a hundred disorders listed in the Diagnostic and Statistical Manual IV-TR. A psychiatric disorder is a disorder that causes problems with thought or emotion. There are six main categories of adult psychiatric disorders: anxiety disorders, mood disorders, psychotic disorders, eating disorders, impulse control and addiction disorders and personality disorders. Many people with psychiatric disorders are able to manage their daily lives independently and without issue. Sometimes, however, the disorder becomes serious enough to warrant a hospitalization, particularly if an individual attempts to cause harm to herself or to others.

Statistics/Demographics

According to the National Institute of Mental Health, in any given year 26.2 percent of adults in the United States meet the diagnostic criteria for some type of mental disorder. A little over 20% of these adults suffer from severe, incapacitating mental illnesses. The Canadian Mental Health Association reports that 20% of Canadians will experience a mental illness in their lifetime. Just over nine percent of adults meet the criteria to be diagnosed with a personality disorder and just over one percent of adults suffer from schizophrenia, a psychotic disorder that causes people to experience hallucinations and delusions.

Prognosis

Suicide is the tenth leading cause of death in both the United States and Canada. Women are more likely to attempt suicide, but men are more likely to complete the act. Currently, the demographic group at the highest risk for suicide is males over the age of 65.

Reasons for Hospitalization

Most people with psychiatric disorders receive treatment from a psychiatrist and/or a therapist on an outpatient basis. Hospitalization is generally used only when a patient is believed to be an immediate threat to herself or to someone else and most hospitalizations last only a few days to a couple of weeks.

Home Care Physical Needs

Most people with psychiatric disorders do not require any assistance with personal care. Acute mental illness can affect people of any age. Schizophrenia and bipolar disorder typically show up during young adulthood. Personality disorders tend to present themselves even earlier. Depression may occur throughout the life cycle, either in response to chemical fluctuations in the brain or to painful life circumstances.

One problem experienced by those who suffer from bipolar disorder is a tendency to stop taking prescribed medication. One reason why individuals stop medications is because they don't like the way a particular medication makes them feel. Another reason why individuals with bipolar disorder stop medication is because they enjoy the manic phase of the disorder. During a manic episode, people have boundless energy and can work on one or many projects for days on end without stopping. Mania can also cause psychotic symptoms, especially delusions of grandeur, and some people with mania get into trouble by running up credit card debt or writing bad checks.

If your loved one speaks to you about stopping medication, strongly encourage her to speak with her doctor or psychiatrist first. If the problem is that your loved one doesn't like the way the medication makes her feel, a trained psychiatrist can adjust the dose, or try another medication. Remind your loved one that it often takes many months after diagnosis or after a flare-up before medications can be regulated.

It helps to know what kinds of side effects your loved one's medications may cause. Antidepressants, for instance, may lead to a lack of interest in sexual activity; antipsychotics may cause a dry mouth and drowsiness. A more serious side effect is involuntary movements, a condition known as tardive dyskinesia. If your loved one experiences involuntary movements while taking an antipsychotic, notify her doctor immediately.

There are some things you can encourage your loved one to do that may help ease her symptoms. Exercise, for instance, can relieve symptoms of depression quite effectively.

Your loved one will also benefit by participating actively in life. This can be hard for a person suffering from depression, who often feels like getting out of bed is a struggle, but studies suggest that once a depressed person becomes involved in an activity, she ends up having a better time than she anticipated.

Home care Emotional Needs

Don't try to "cheer up" a depressed loved one or tell her to "snap out of it." She would if she could.

Having any type of psychiatric disorder, but especially depression, is a risk factor for suicide. If you suspect your loved one is thinking about harming herself, ask her directly. You won't put ideas in her head. In fact, if she is feeling suicidal, talking about it is a safe way to discharge the feelings without acting upon them.

Mental health professionals generally deem the risk factor for suicide to be low if the person has only vague thoughts of wanting to die, expresses conflict between wanting to die and wanting to live, does not have a specific plan and has no means of suicide at her disposal.

The risk factor increases if your loved one has a specific plan for killing herself and if the means are readily available to her.

> **Resource Corner:** A suicide threat is a serious issue. If you're not sure whether or not a suicide threat is serious, call the person's psychiatrist or therapist. If they are not available, call 911 and have her transported to an emergency room where she can be examined by a mental health professional.

CHAPTER TWENTY-FOUR
Transitioning from Hospital to Home

Bringing an individual home from the hospital, especially if the individual's care needs have increased, can seem daunting. Taking the following steps will help ensure that you are as prepared as possible for your loved one's homecoming.

1. Meet with the Health Care Team to Discuss Your Loved One's New Needs

If your loved one lived alone prior to the hospitalization, you need to seriously consider whether she can continue to do so. If your loved one needs a few days or weeks before she feels secure in returning to living alone, perhaps she could be referred to an inpatient rehabilitation unit to regain strength and encourage independence. One option for individuals who wish to remain at home but still require rehabilitation is to to hire a private duty caregiver to assist in activities of daily living and have the rehabilitation team come to the home a few times a week.

If living alone is no longer an option for your loved one, take some time to think before committing yourself as a full, or part-time caregiver. How will your new role affect your work, your relationships with your family and your own health?

You may decide that your loved one's needs are too great and that you are not in a position to become a primary caregiver. There is no shame in making that decision. Once you have made it, you, your loved one and the discharge team can discuss other options, such as moving in with another family member who is in a position to care for your loved one, hiring a private duty home care caregiver or moving to a nursing home or an assisted living facility.

2. Ask Friends/Family for Help

You may decide that you are capable of caring for your loved one at home. This certainly doesn't mean that you have to do everything on your own. Often, when an elderly parent needs increased care, one family member is left "holding the bag." To avoid finding yourself in this position, be assertive when it comes to asking for help. Be pleasant but direct when you make a request. "I need to get away for a few hours on Saturday. Could you come over and stay with Dad from noon until five?" or "I need a caregiver to help me with Uncle George's baths. If all of us could agree to pitch in $25.00 per month that should cover the cost."

3. Prepare Your Home

Make your home as safe as possible. This is especially important if the individual suffers from Alzheimer's disease or another form of dementia and is not aware of basic safety issues.

First, go through the house and remove all the clutter from the floor. Check to make sure there are no electric cords stretching across a room or hallway. It's also a good idea to remove throw rugs from any room your loved one is likely to enter. Throw rugs may look attractive, but they can easily get bunched up under your loved one's feet and cause a fall.

Another way to help prevent falls is installing sturdy grab bars by the toilet and inside the bathtub or shower. Investing in a tub bench, available at most retail pharmacies for a reasonable price, can further reduce the risk of falling.

If your loved one suffers from dementia, wandering may be a problem, especially in a new environment. Install tricky locks and/or alarms on all the doors leading to the outside. Prevent scalding injuries by lowering the temperature on the water thermostat.

Finally, make sure all medications or other toxic products your loved one might accidentally ingest are safely locked away.

4. Arrange for Delivery of Medical Equipment

The individual may be discharged from the hospital needing special equipment such as an oxygen concentrator, a wheelchair or a hospital bed. The hospital social worker can fax the doctor's order and the discharged patient's insurance information to an appropriate medical equipment supplier to facilitate the delivery of the equipment to the home.

The supplier usually plans to deliver the medical equipment a day or so before discharge to ensure that it is all set up and ready to go when the patient arrives home.

Take a few minutes and think about where the equipment will best fit in your house. If you decide to put the hospital bed in a guest room, for instance, what will you do with the bed that is already there? People who deliver medical equipment are glad to set up the equipment and train you in its use, but it is not their responsibility to help you disassemble or move other pieces of furniture.

One last step you can take is making sure that a wheelchair fits through the doorways of rooms they will need to access, such as the bathroom or the bedroom.

5. Coordinate In-Home Services

Find out from the discharge planner if the doctor has recommended Medicare-covered services like home health care or hospice. Make sure the discharge planner has all of the patient's insurance information so that he or she can locate a provider who will work with your insurance company.

If the discharge planning team does not believe your loved one would benefit from home health care or from hospice, consider hiring a caregiver from a private duty home care agency, especially if the individual requires a lot of physical assistance or if you are not comfortable helping him with intimate tasks like toileting or bathing.

Most health insurance plans do not cover what they term "custodial care," but some long term care insurance plans do cover the cost of these services. If your loved one has long term care insurance, speak with his agent to see if the insurance plan will help.

The state or county where your loved one resides may also assist with the cost of private duty care, especially if your loved one can show financial need.

Most frequently, though, your loved one will need to pay for private duty care out of his own pocket. Work with the company to arrange a schedule your loved one can afford while still ensuring that both you and he get the assistance you need.

6. Arrange Transportation Home from the Hospital

In many cases, you will be able to bring your loved one home in your own car. If, however, your loved one must be transported in a wheelchair, or if he is too weak to sit up for a car trip, you may need to hire a wheelchair van, an ambulance or a home care agency to bring your loved one home. The hospital social worker or the discharge planner can help you arrange alternate transportation, although your loved one will have to pay for it. Note that many wheelchair van companies insist that their driver be paid before he or she provides the transportation; most ambulance companies will send you a bill.

7. Expect the Unexpected

While going home after a hospitalization is a joyous, triumphant occasion for some, it can be a daunting, stress-provoking time for others. Especially in cases where an individual's physical condition has changed drastically, it is quite common for the individual and his loved ones to struggle with anger, uncertainty and depression. Maintaining a positive but realistic outlook is important. Work with the discharge team to devise an organized post-discharge plan and use the pervious chapters of this book to educate yourself on life after hospitalization.

Offer your loved one as much support and understanding as you can while he makes the adjustment to his new circumstances. At the same time, remember to stay in close touch with your own support system of friends, family, clergy, etc. The transition from hospital to home care can be a challenge for everyone involved. Try not to worry if it all seems too complex and frightening at first—humans are incredibly resilient and able to adapt. You and your loved one are both exploring uncharted territory. Trust that you will, eventually, get used to your new reality and establish a routine that works for both of you. It just takes some time and patience.

CHAPTER TWENTY-FIVE
Summary

Although it is impossible to plan for every single situation that may arise after a hospitalization, this book explores some of the most common concerns patients and their caregivers face when making the transition from hospital to home.

We hope you've found all the information within these pages to be valuable, but if you take away only one thought from the book, let it be this: The hospitalization experience is already stressful enough that you will want to use whatever resources are available to use for the transition home. Trying to be a full-time caregiver when you have a long list of competing responsibilities will not only endanger your own health but also increase your risk of burnout and decrease the likelihood that you will be able to continue providing care for your loved one.

Whether assistance comes in the form of family, friends, neighbors, people you know from church, or professional support from a private duty home care company like Home Care Assistance, ask for help!

Ask now, even if you don't think you need help yet. You may be surprised to realize how much you enjoy having a few hours to yourself. Besides, if you wait until you are too mentally and physically exhausted to seek help, it may be too late to salvage the caregiving situation.

Physically write into your daily schedule a fifteen to thirty minute time frame when you will focus on yourself. Perhaps you can set this time to coincide with your loved one's naps, her time in adult daycare, or the hour or two a day when she goes to a rehabilitation clinic. During your "me-time," consider the following activities:

- Read a chapter or two of a novel by your favorite author
- Pray or meditate
- Listen to your favorite music
- Walk around the block
- Snuggle up with a pet
- Spend time with someone you love
- Make a list of everything—big and small—that you've accomplished in the last week
- Take a hot bath or a shower
- Watch a funny movie or sitcom and let yourself laugh out loud
- Take a power nap

These are just a few suggestions. The point is that the better you care for yourself, the better you'll be able to care for your loved one.

Finally, always remember that there are resources at hand to help you with your loved one's care. You may have to look hard for them, and you may have to ask for their help, but they do exist. Tapping into these resources is a great way to improve your loved one's quality of life and your own as well. If you would like to discuss your situation with a care manager or learn more about arranging home care services, visit **www.HomeCareAssistance.com** or call (toll-free) **1-866-4-LiveIn** or **1-866-454-8346**.

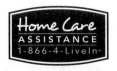

About Home Care Assistance

Our mission at Home Care Assistance is to change the way the world ages. We provide older adults with quality care that enables them to live happier, healthier lives at home. Our services are distinguished by the caliber of our caregivers, the responsiveness of our staff and our expertise in Live-In care. We embrace a positive, balanced approach to aging centered on the evolving needs of older adults.

- **Live-In Experts.** We specialize in around the clock care to help seniors live well at home.

- **Available 24/7.** Care managers are on call for clients and their families, even during nights and weekends.

- **High Caliber Caregivers.** We hire only 1 in 25 applicants and provide ongoing training and supervision.

- **Balanced Care.** Our unique approach to care promotes healthy mind, body and spirit.

- **No Long Term Contracts.** Use our services only as long as you're 100% satisfied.

- **A Trusted Partner.** We're honored to be Preferred Providers for professionals in both the medical and senior communities.

- **Peace of Mind.** Independent industry surveys place our client satisfaction rate at 97%.

Author Biographies

Kathy N. Johnson, PhD, CMC is a Certified Geriatric Care Manager and Chief Executive Officer of Home Care Assistance. A recognized leader in senior care, she holds a Doctorate in Psychology from the Illinois Institute of Technology.

James H. Johnson, PhD is a licensed clinical psychologist and Chairman of Home Care Assistance. He is the former department chair of the Virginia Consortium for Professional Psychology and the award-winning author of nine books. He holds a Doctorate in Psychology from the University of Minnesota.

Lily Sarafan, MS is President and Chief Operating Officer of Home Care Assistance. She has been featured as an industry expert by more than 100 media outlets. She holds Masters and Bachelors degrees from Stanford University.

NOTES

NOTES

NOTES

NOTES

NOTES

NOTES